The Palliative Approach:
A Resource for Healthcare Workers

Other books from M&K include

My Health, My Faith, My Culture:
A guide for healthcare practitioners
ISBN: 9781905539802

Nurses and Their Patients:
Informing practice through psychodynamic insights
ISBN: 9781905539314

Spiritual Assessment in Healthcare Practice
ISBN: 9781905539277

The Clinician's Guide to Chronic Disease Management for Long-Term Conditions:
A cognitive-behavioural approach
ISBN: 9781905539154

Therapy Skills for Healthcare:
An introduction to brief psychological techniques
ISBN: 9781905539581

Contents

Figures

About the author

Erica Cameron-Taylor trained as a General Practitioner before undertaking advanced training in palliative care. She now works as a staff specialist and is a conjoint senior lecturer at the University of Newcastle, New South Wales, Australia. Her particular interests are integrating palliative care into generalist care paradigms, palliative care in dementia and medical education.

Introduction

This book is not a medical text, nor is it a text describing advanced nursing practice for the care of terminally ill and dying patients. It does not deal with complex patients requiring the specialist care of tertiary inpatient palliative care units. There are myriad other excellent texts that serve this purpose. It is intended instead to provide a simple and commonsense introduction to the care of patients in the generalist setting for whom a palliative approach is deemed appropriate.

Many of these patients may be living at home or in care homes, and many may be months or even years away from the terminal phase of illness. It is hoped that this text will provide an initial resource for healthcare professionals to give them an understanding of, and a competence in, the provision of quality-of-life and comfort-focused care. Its development has arisen from the questions and concerns of many students, staff members and families, many of whom have said '…but I just don't know what to do or say'.

The medications used to treat specific symptoms will vary between countries, units and care settings. The information regarding medications in this text is brief and provided only in order to illustrate points of care. It does not replace competent medical review and should not be relied upon for prescribing.

This book is intended to provide a simple initial tool to guide the optimisation of care for a rapidly growing population of patients for whom the diagnostic and cure-focused aims of contemporary medicine have less to offer.

Note: Bracketed references in the text refer to publications listed in 'Further reading and references' on page 111.

Acknowledgement
Thanks are due to the staff of the Department of Palliative Care at Calvary Mater, Newcastle, New South Wales.

Chapter 1

What is palliative care?

No area of medicine has received as much attention as palliative care – in the sense of workshops conducted and articles written. Work still continues on finding the best name for this type of care, with various services around the globe using terms such as 'hospice care' and 'supportive care' among others.

The fact that palliative care cannot be defined by an organ (unlike cardiology or nephrology), by the chronology of a specific disease, or by the geographic boundary of a single patient, creates the need for a complex definition. Even the World Health Organisation (WHO) had trouble, and the wording they ended up with hints at consensus by a *big* panel!

The current WHO definition of 'palliative care' is (www.who.int/cancer/palliative/definition/en/):

> **an approach that improves the quality of life of patients and their families facing the problems associated with life-threatening illness, through the prevention and relief of suffering by means of early identification and impeccable assessment and treatment of pain and other problems, physical, psychosocial and spiritual.**

Palliative care:
- Provides relief from pain and other distressing symptoms;
- Affirms life and regards dying as a normal process;
- Intends neither to hasten or postpone death;
- Integrates the psychological and spiritual aspects of patient care;
- Offers a support system to help patients live as actively as possible until death;
- Offers a support system to help the family cope during the patient's illness and in their own bereavement;
- Uses a team approach to address the needs of patients and their families, including bereavement counselling, if indicated;

1

- Will enhance quality of life, and may also positively influence the course of illness;
- Is applicable early in the course of illness, in conjunction with other therapies that are intended to prolong life, such as chemotherapy or radiation therapy, and includes those investigations needed to better understand and manage distressing clinical complications.

No other medical specialty has such a long definition and certainly no other requires multiple bullet points! It is difficult to avoid the feeling that palliative medicine is still desperate to ensure that it is taken seriously.

The cumbersome WHO definition has led many units and services to develop their own, simpler version. The definition used by the unit in which I practise is:

Palliative care is the integrated and multidisciplinary assessment, management, support and care of patients, their families and carers, who are living with active, progressive and far-advanced disease for whom cure is no longer an option, prognosis is limited, and where quality of life is the central concern. Palliative care is holistic, patient-focused care and support is continued into the bereavement phase.

Not that long ago, for many patients a referral to 'palliative care' represented 'being thrown on the scrapheap', and for many doctors it represented defeat. Palliative care was care that was delivered when everything else had been tried. It was simple and kind, but it also represented failure: the failure of a healthcare system devoted to cure, and the failure of a body that could no longer recover and be rehabilitated. However, the aims and spirit that developed palliative care were very different from that dismal viewpoint, and the particular benefits of this type of care are beginning to be seen as appropriate in many different settings.

The 'traditional' recipient of palliative care is the cancer patient who has reached the end of their curative treatments such as chemotherapy and radiotherapy and who now relies on symptom control measures to provide an optimised quality of life and as much comfort as possible in the terminal phase. However, in recent years, the profile of patients being accepted onto palliative care services has expanded from exclusively cancer patients to a greater variety of conditions including end-stage organ failure and neurodegenerative diseases such as motor neurone disease.

Services differ on their specific criteria for acceptance into a palliative care programme. Some services happily accept patients with severe dementia, chronic obstructive airway (pulmonary) disease or severe stroke, whilst others are more reluctant to take such a broad spectrum of patients. Many palliative care services operate both inpatient and community outreach services and may have different admission criteria for each.

Services that provide a consultation service for other medical specialties may see all patients referred to them and give advice, but may only accept a proportion of those patients as 'palliative care patients'. In many areas, 'palliative care' is now instituted in tandem with continuing active treatment such as chemotherapy. As the disease progresses, the care focus gradually shifts from being predominantly cure-focused to being totally palliative. Contemporary palliative care recognises that the transition to a palliative approach is difficult for the patient, the family, the carers, and the treating team, and that gradual introduction and transition is preferable to sudden change.

In the last decade, palliative medicine has become a medical speciality in its own right, and tertiary centres manage patients with difficult and complex symptoms who cannot be optimally managed in the community or on general wards. These centres aim to provide education and support for all healthcare staff who look after patients for whom the focus of care is no longer simply cure.

The modern concept that medicine is a 'curative art' is just that – very modern. For most of medicine's history, the best that could be done was to alleviate symptoms and provide comfort. The opportunity to 'cure' has only come with the advent of agents to fight infection and the skill to perform specific curative surgical techniques. As medical advancement continued at a rapid pace, the focus of medicine shifted from providing care and comfort to the contemporary aims of scientific, evidence-based investigation, diagnosis and treatment aimed at cure. There were always places that cared for the dying, but, as modern medicine gained momentum, care for the dying became a low priority. Even today, it is much easier to raise money to buy expensive equipment to treat a very rare disease that affects the young than it is to provide care for the dying. This sheds an interesting light on priorities in modern society, given that we all have a 100% chance of dying in this lifetime!

The modern hospice movement really began in England in the late 1960s and 1970s, inspired by the work of the indomitable Dame Cicely Saunders at St Christopher's in London, whose dedication, insight and passion still informs contemporary palliative care (Saunders 1990).

The Liverpool Care Pathway for the Dying Patient was developed in the UK in the late 1990s. This protocol has since been modified by centres across the globe to provide a framework that enables nurses and doctors to optimise the management of the terminal phase for their inpatients. However, outside acute hospitals, there is a great need for guidance on terminal phase management. As a relatively new specialty, palliative care is perhaps still 'finding its place' in many centres but the approaches it offers are being rapidly integrated into the care of an ever-wider patient population.

Not everyone who dies requires the expertise of a tertiary or specialist palliative care service. Specialist units are used for patients who have complex needs and problematic symptoms, and particularly for patients with escalating opiate requirements. These patients are not the ones referred to in this book. However, all patients will die at some stage, and for many of those patients death is expected. For these patients, and their carers, the palliative approach has much to offer and they are the focus of this book.

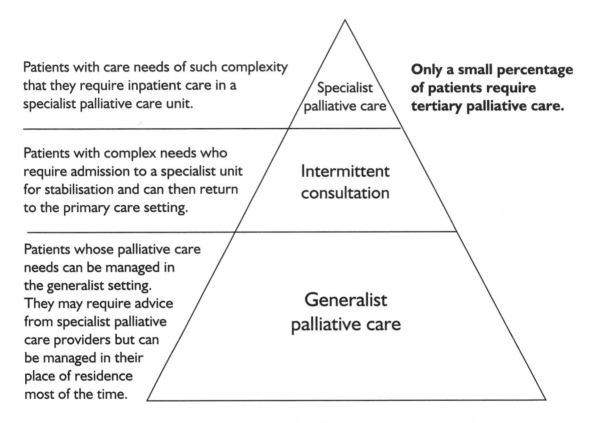

Patients with care needs of such complexity that they require inpatient care in a specialist palliative care unit.

Specialist palliative care

Only a small percentage of patients require tertiary palliative care.

Patients with complex needs who require admission to a specialist unit for stabilisation and can then return to the primary care setting.

Intermittent consultation

Patients whose palliative care needs can be managed in the generalist setting. They may require advice from specialist palliative care providers but can be managed in their place of residence most of the time.

Generalist palliative care

Figure 1.1 *What type of palliative care is required?*

Chapter 2
The palliative approach

In simple terms, the palliative approach is a way of thinking about quality-focused care rather than cure-focused care. It is also a term used to gently distinguish those patients whose symptoms can be managed in a general setting from those who require the specialist care implied by the medical term 'palliative care'. The distinction is often an arbitrary one. This book therefore focuses on optimising the provision of supportive and palliative care for all patients for whom death is expected (be that in days, weeks, months or even years), who do not require the expertise of a specialist intensive palliative care unit.

Having to decide when and whether a palliative approach is appropriate often involves complex and emotive issues. The best scenario is that such a decision evolves organically, rather than being suddenly imposed in a crisis. This organic approach informs many of the assessment tools being introduced in care facilities for the elderly and it is a core value in living wills (also known as advance care directives).

However, in some cases, palliative care has to be provided as an acute response. Such situations might include, for example, deciding not to offer neurosurgical intervention in the case of sudden intracerebral haemorrhage, or deciding to provide comfort-only care in a case of sudden fulminant sepsis despite intravenous antibiotics. Instances of such acute palliative care intervention, and their complex ethical and legal dimensions, are beyond the scope of this book (see Further reading and references, page 111).

For most patients, death is heralded long before it actually occurs and it is for these patients that the palliative approach holds great potential benefit. But we must, of course, guard against oversimplification. The 'palliative approach' is often viewed as a philosophy that guides the levels of investigation and intervention that a certain patient wishes to receive. For instance, it may be cited as a reason for not transferring a patient from a care facility for the elderly to an acute hospital, for commencing oral rather than intramuscular or intravenous antibiotics in the face of a worsening infection, or for not considering surgical intervention. However, it is important for a palliative approach to remain patient-centred from the outset and not become a vehicle for other, veiled, agendas.

It is the duty of every healthcare professional to consider not just every patient, but also every episode in the care of each patient. For example, wanting to pursue the palliative approach in the care of an 85-year-old man with moderate dementia does not negate the fact that the single best way to manage his pain due to a fracture may be orthopaedic intervention. On the other hand, it may be entirely appropriate to use the palliative approach to prevent the same patient's transfer away from his familiar surroundings to an acute hospital during his terminal phase, but high-dose antibiotic therapy may still be the optimal treatment for painful parotiditis (salivary gland infection).

No 'blanket directive' can ever encompass every situation a patient may face. The benefits of a palliative approach must therefore be vigilantly assessed at each new step in a patient's journey, rather than simply at the outset. A particular care path must never be used to legitimise non-patient-focused agendas such as the need to deal with shortages of staff or resources, over-complex paperwork or institutional politics.

The opinion of competent patients, and their family members or designated advocates or surrogate decision-makers, should be regularly sought to ensure that no changes have occurred and there is no new desire to pursue more active treatment, even if the care team members believe that this would be futile. The patient and their family have the right to change their minds. They also, once fully informed, have the right to make the 'wrong' decision! At every step along the way, the central question/s should be asked: 'Is this what the patient wants?' and/or 'Is this the best way to optimise quality of life, comfort and dignity for this patient at this time?' Only when the patient's best interests lie at the heart of each decision can we be sure that our clinical duty of care (and our ethical and moral responsibility to the patient) is at one with the care approach we are using, palliative or otherwise.

It is impossible to create a list of all patients for whom the palliative approach may be appropriate. To consider only the dying ignores many other patients for whom palliative care can be of great benefit. In general terms, patients who fall into the following categories should be reviewed:

- Patients in the final weeks, days or hours of life
- Patients with advanced or metastatic malignancy who have no further treatment options or who have declined further treatment

- Patients with malignancy who are approaching a transition from curative to palliative care
- Patients with symptomatic deterioration during maximal medical treatment for heart, liver or lung failure
- Patients with end-stage renal disease, or dialysis patients with declining response to dialysis or who express a desire to cease treatment
- Patients with advanced or end-stage dementia
- The 'oldest old'
- Patients with complex co-morbidities whose quality of life and function continues to decline despite repeated intervention
- Patients with incurable, far advanced and/or progressive neurological compromise
- Patients who have been unable to recover cognitive and physical function following an event such as a cerebral vascular accident or a myocardial infarct
- Patients with complex care needs such as those who have profound intellectual and physical disabilities

When considering which patients are suitable for a palliative approach to care, the following broad categories should be explored:
- Patient wishes
- Family and carer wishes
- Medical issues
- Disease stage
- Life stage

Patient wishes

If the patient is mentally competent and – after effective discussion – does not agree with the adoption of the palliative approach, this should be clearly documented and the 'normal' pattern of care continued without further delay. The issue may, of course, be revisited but the statutes of informed consent, patient autonomy and confidentiality that inform all clinical practice are just as relevant when discussing the issue of palliative care as they are in other clinical domains.

All palliative care practitioners have had the experience of arriving to review a patient after a request for consultation has been received – only to find that the patient is not only unaware of the review but is unaware of the proposed withdrawal of curative treatment. Any referral to palliative care, and any discussion of the palliative approach, requires the current care team to carefully consider the needs of the patient and their family as they reach this new stage in the illness journey. For many people, any mention of the word 'palliative' immediately conjures up an image of a hospice from which they believe no one emerges alive. The role of contemporary palliative care in supportive management and symptom control, often for many months or years, is not well understood. Appropriate and sensitive discussion by the treating team, the provision of accessible education, allowing time for information to be absorbed, and carefully timed referral are all important elements that can help ensure that palliative care review will have the hoped-for outcome.

Careless referral and poor communication in the initial stages can create barriers of confusion, fear, resentment, misunderstanding and alienation, which can lead to a refusal to accept palliative care advice. This, in turn, can have a profound and detrimental effect on the comfort and dignity of death.

Difficult discussions around issues such as the 'Not for Resuscitation' (NFR/DNR) orders that are used in the palliative approach are dealt with elsewhere in this book but it is important to note here that informed consent requires patients to understand the issue being discussed. It is therefore imperative that the clinical team members are able to simply and effectively discuss the concept of palliative care with their patient. This may take some time. Often, a couple of brief interventions are more effective than one long discussion, particularly with elderly, distressed or very unwell patients.

Before beginning any discussion, consider carefully the situation of this particular patient at this time. There is no generic form for such a conversation. The issues for a 97-year-old care home resident with breast cancer are by no means the same as those for a 40-year-old mother living at home with two teenage daughters, even though the two women may have the same disease and the same life expectancy. The following suggestions are therefore guidelines only.

1. Introduce the topic

'Mary, today I want to have a talk to you about your healthcare and about planning for the future…'

'Tom, you've been through a really rough time recently and I want to talk to you about how we can perhaps make things easier…'

'I'm sorry that all Dr Little's tests showed the cancer has spread, John, but I'm hoping we can have a chat about things we might be able to do to help…'

'Ethel, Sara and I are quite concerned about you and we want to understand a bit more about how you feel about what's been going on…'

2. Define the palliative approach

'Bill, sometimes when we know there is a problem we can't cure, we decide to focus healthcare on comfort and quality of life. I think that, for you, this may be beneficial. In this type of healthcare we concentrate on care that increases your comfort, but doesn't focus as much on repeated tests or procedures that don't really help you feel better. You know we can't cure you, but there's still a lot we can do.'

3. Define treatment issues

'Toby, I need to ask you whether, if you got another serious chest infection that wasn't getting better with tablets, you'd want us to transfer you to hospital again and use antibiotics through the vein, or whether you'd like to stay here and just be kept comfortable?'

'Laura, if the effects of the stroke get worse and you can't eat, or if your breathing is worse, are you happy to stay here and let us care for you and keep you comfortable, or do you want us to send you back to hospital?'

'Mick, you know that, with your health being as it is, something could happen at any time. If you did become more unwell, is it your wish that we concentrate on your comfort, or do you want to be sent straight to hospital?'

In many cases providing a brief explanation of the contrast between the palliative approach and routine care is helpful. You could say something like:

'Often what we do when someone becomes more unwell is send them off for tests, and perhaps send them to hospital, in case some procedure can be carried out. We're wondering if, because your health is so poor, you might prefer to stay at home and have comfort care in that situation. What do you think?'

4. Summarise the patient's wishes

'So, Tom, let me make sure I know exactly what your wishes are: you don't want us to try and resuscitate you if your heart stops, but you do want antibiotics if you get an infection, but just don't want to have to go to hospital. If things get to the point that the end of your life is close you are happy to stay here and be kept comfortable. Is that right?'

It is important to reiterate the concept of autonomy. For some patients, a situation where they are confined to a wheelchair, reliant on nursing care and needing dialysis twice a week could lead them to feel a great desire to embrace the palliative approach and accept natural death, but others would be grateful for each extra day of life and would wish to pursue life-sustaining treatment for as long as possible. The care team should not advocate either approach, but it *is* their role to inform and educate, to respect the patient's decision, and to ensure that any decision the patient makes is free from coercion.

We must also remember that many people have determinedly stated 'if I can't look after myself and I'm no use to anyone then I want to be allowed to die' but have subsequently realised that they won't 'just die'. Their condition will fluctuate, rather than following a predictable course, and their concept of what constitutes human worth may change when they are actually in the state that they previously considered 'useless'. For all these reasons, living wills or advance care directives (whilst valuable) never negate the need for repeated review.

The aim of the palliative approach must never be 'the scrapheap'. A great deal of research has shown that the desire for hastened death frequently relates not to severe pain or distressing symptoms, but instead to feeling worthless, useless and a burden. The issue of euthanasia is discussed elsewhere in this book but any patient who voices a desire for comfort-only care due to feelings of worthlessness, despair, loneliness or guilt must receive competent psychiatric review as a matter of urgency.

5. Reassure and revisit

'Thank you for talking to me about all that. I want to assure you that this new plan simply means that your comfort is now our number one focus. Do you have any questions or worries about anything we've talked about? If you change your mind we can alter things at any time. I might come back in a few days to just check with you if that's OK...'

'Thanks, Jacob. It's really important that we know what your wishes are and I'll make sure I record everything we've spoken about in the notes. I just want to reassure you that your decision to have the ambulance called straight away if you have another stroke is respected by all of us, and we'll do our best to make sure that happens. If you have any worries or questions, you can talk to me or John at any time.'

Family and carer wishes

The wishes of family and carers are easy to manage when they align with our own wishes and those of our patients, and a cause of much distress when they don't! The family determined to pursue active, aggressive and frequently onerous treatment despite evidence of its inappropriateness is more common than the family who request comfort-only care when there is an effective option, but both exist. Examples of the former may include: the very close and intertwined child, for example the daughter who has spent her adult life caring for her mother at home; the adult 'child' who has lived overseas for many years and has returned to an elderly parent whose health has deteriorated in their absence; the family member who has a position of authority and influence in their work but feels ineffectual and threatened in the face of serious illness; and the family member who has suffered another significant loss recently, or has experienced poor resolution of previous grief.

There are several issues to consider when reviewing the wishes of the family and carers. Firstly, do they have the patient's best interests at heart and are they right? Is there something that has been missed? The second consideration is to ensure that the family members are carefully informed about all the issues. If the therapeutic relationship is strained, this may require you to enlist the help of someone outside the team. Many supposed disagreements about the care path are actually a result of poor understanding or a lack of information. A carer may have been shown a pathology report and scan results detailing widespread metastatic disease but that does not mean they understand all the implications. Many people either forget or misinterpret much of the medical information they are given. Careful discussion in simple terms is a vital first step in resolving any disagreement.

This sounds simple but it is a skill that requires practice and confidence and is not well taught at medical school. Complex medical language can be used to shield us from uncomfortable, emotive concepts such as mortality, grief, suffering and loss. It may be valuable for nursing staff, for example, to discuss the information with the medical practitioner, or to be present during discussions with the patient and family, and then serve as an 'interpreter'. Care must always be taken to provide accurate information and to resist the temptation to present opinion and intuition as medical fact.

In any disagreement with carers, the patient's views and feelings must be our first priority. If the patient is competent and willing to express their opinion, their own wishes obviously over-rule those of their carer. If the patient is not mentally competent, then it may be necessary to consider resorting to the offices of the Public Guardianship Board or other authorities. It is situations where family dynamics lead to a competent patient not expressing their wishes, or changing their mind depending on which family member is present, that cause the greatest concern.

In these cases, it is important to remember that it is not the role of the caring team to try to heal a dysfunctional family. It is their role to care for the patient. A pattern of interaction that may seem 'pathological' to the healthcare team may be the only pattern that a particular family knows. These ways of behaving can be so entrenched that the family has no insight into the issues and a compromise solution may be the best outcome possible.

Organising a family meeting, ensuring that all the important stakeholders (including the patient!) and a variety of clinical staff are present, is often an important step in managing these situations. The disease story, the current issues and concerns, and the opinions of the patient, care team and the family, should all be reviewed, with the aim of returning responsibility for achieving consensus to the family. Careful, accurate and contemporaneous documentation of these meetings is vital.

Referral to social workers, pastoral care, psychology or psychiatry services should be considered when there are significant concerns.

Medical issues

For the majority of patients, there are well-defined medical issues that lead them towards a palliative mode of care. It is imperative that there is documented evidence of the medical situation, and evidence of treatments provided in the past. No patient should ever be 'presumed' to be palliative without the sighting of evidence such as histology reports, scan results, specialist letters, discharge summaries and functional assessments.

Disease stage

The concept of disease stage is closely related to the ability of the patient, carers and family to accept the fact that intensive medical care now has little to offer. Many people watching closely as a loved one deteriorates forget how the present situation fits into the overall disease story and therefore perspective can be lost.

Instead of saying '*Well, as you know, Harry's got prostate cancer and now it's in his liver and they've done all they can,*' it's much more useful to meet with the patient and family and summarise the disease story:

> 'As you know, Harry's had a long journey with his prostate cancer and I'd just like to summarise it for us all. He was diagnosed with prostate cancer 10 years ago and had radiation treatment. All was well for a few years but then his prostate marker levels went up again and he started on hormone treatment. This helped for a year or so but, unfortunately, the cancer continued to grow and in the middle of last year scans showed that it had spread to his bones. Harry's had other problems too, including heart disease and diabetes, and recently he has become much weaker and more frail, and a scan has

shown cancer in his liver. There is nothing more that can be done to slow the cancer but there is still a lot we can do to make sure that Harry is comfortable.'

Life stage

The palliative approach fits naturally at the end of a long life when the normal aging process, perhaps augmented by a specific disease, has already started to lead towards death. However, when the end of a patient's life is approaching at a younger age the issues are very different.

As medical care and living standards have improved, life expectancy has changed, and most people now assume that they and their loved ones will live into their eighties or longer. For example, in 2011 the Bureau of Statistics in Australia quoted the average life expectancy for females as 83.76 years and for males 78.29 years.

The special issues of paediatric palliative care and the care of terminally ill young adults (Wolfe, Hinds & Sourkes 2011) are outside the scope of this book but most families today will feel that the approaching death of a person in their forties, fifties and even sixties is 'too soon'. Any disruption to the natural order of parents pre-deceasing their children obviously adds greatly to the emotional burden of this situation. The fact that people are training for longer, staying in the workforce longer and having children later also means that many families are facing the loss of a person who, fifty years ago, might have been a loved one and parent, but is now a parent, a child and breadwinner as well.

For some people who feel they are 'dying before their time', the palliative approach will never be acceptable. Their right to strive to stay alive to their last breath must be respected. For others, a palliative mode of care can provide comfort and dignity and allow important conversations to occur and legacy building to be achieved.

Any discussion of a transition to palliative care must therefore take into account all the available medical information, the disease stage and the life stage of the patient, and the wishes of all the major stakeholders. The patient's wishes must remain at the centre of any discussion. If decision-making is deferred to a patient advocate, careful communication is the cornerstone in achieving an optimal outcome. For the vast majority of patients for whom the information in this book is intended, there is no need to make a final decision in a short timeframe. Allowing information to be assimilated and digested, and providing an opportunity for review and discussion, is often a therapeutic intervention in itself.

Multidisciplinary care

Effective palliative care requires a multidisciplinary approach. It is impossible to over-estimate the benefit of competent and effective physiotherapy, occupational therapy, pastoral care and social work. There are very few patients who do not respond positively to the involvement of these allied health professionals. It is best to access allied health professionals as part of a team but, if this is not possible, independent allied health practitioner advice can be sought on a case-by-case basis and integrated into the care of a particular patient.

For example, massage therapists can offer significant help in relation to pain and psychological well-being. Any symptom is made worse by sadness, loneliness and fear, and services provided by pastoral care workers, volunteers, social workers, grief counsellors, religious personnel and psychologists can therefore help make the difference between a poor outcome and an optimal one.

Occupational therapists

Occupational therapists work with patients and families to ensure that patients are able to live as fully and independently as possible. They respond to patients' needs and assist in the development of strategies, goals and care plans that reflect each individual's preferences.

Occupational therapists can support patients by providing specialised equipment and tailoring activities and education to their needs and wishes. Central to the work of all the allied health disciplines is the recognition that each individual has unique experiences, goals and priorities. An occupational therapist can assist a patient if they are not able to participate in leisure activities or they are having difficulty completing everyday tasks such as showering or transferring from a bed to a chair, or they are experiencing discomfort when sitting or lying down. In inpatient settings, occupational therapists can provide invaluable assistance with the treatment and prevention of pressure sores and muscle contractures.

Physiotherapists

Physiotherapists are experts in movement. They can design a specific exercise plan or teach carers assisted movement techniques that can help the patient regain or preserve joint mobility, avoid muscle contracture, improve function and assist in pain management. They can facilitate a patient's ability to remain mobile and can institute techniques to maintain independence.

The provision of specialist chest physiotherapy is an integral part of the management of several chronic lung conditions. Physiotherapists also play a vital role in managing lymphoedema and can advise on the use of transcutaneous electrical nerve stimulation (TENS) machines and massage therapy. They often work in conjunction with an occupational therapist to optimise the quality of life and functional capacity of individual patients.

Pharmacists

Pharmacists provide information about medications for both patients and carers. They can help simplify medication regimes and provide support for medical staff in situations of complex management requiring multiple medications. Their advice is particularly valuable when it comes to avoiding unwanted side-effects in the context of multi-drug regimes.

Pastoral care staff

Pastoral care staff can assist patients, families and carers to manage the complex emotional and spiritual issues that surround serious illness and approaching death. The importance of these practitioners has grown as the influence of traditional organised religion has lessened in society. However, it is important to remember that even patients with strong support from a religious community can benefit greatly from pastoral care support. The expertise of these practitioners continues to be of great value through the bereavement phase.

Social workers

Social workers can often assist with practical issues such as finance, guardianship, power-of-attorney documentation, advance care directives and accessing services. Social work practitioners play a vital part in arranging care placement for the elderly and they can help family members access any benefits to which they may be entitled. They also have an important role in the proactive provision of support for families who are identified as vulnerable.

Diversional therapists

In New Zealand and Australia, there are diversional therapists who can offer patients and their families the opportunity to engage in a range of activities to maintain interest and social contact and also facilitate legacy building. For example, the opportunity for a young father to record a CD of favourite bedtime stories for his child, or for a grandmother to compile a recipe book for a much-loved granddaughter, can often be of more benefit to a patient than any medication.

Research staff

Research staff may become involved if patients enter a clinical trial. Patients in the palliative phase of care form a unique group and the need for evidence-based medicine is no less for them than it is for other patient groups. Whilst some staff may have mixed feelings about the idea of clinical trials in palliative care, trials are increasing in number and many patients find joining one of them a rewarding and affirming undertaking.

When to refer and how to assimilate allied health advice

Allied health intervention is almost always beneficial. However, concerns can sometimes arise about recognising when referral is needed, and finding a way to integrate the resulting advice.

The more appropriate question would be when *not* to refer. When any patient starts on a palliative approach pathway, physiotherapy and occupational therapy referrals should be routine, if possible. There is no need to wait until an incident occurs. Most patients who are referred to a physiotherapist with, for example, a rotator cuff tear, or to an occupational therapist after problems getting dressed independently, would have benefited greatly from review months, if not years, previously.

The allied health practitioner's ability to provide rapid and effective intervention for any patient is greatly enhanced if the practitioner is already familiar with that person's baseline function. The practitioner's assessments of movement and function are vital components in everything from discharge planning and equipment provision to service delivery. The ability to compare professional functional assessments over time gives the care team invaluable and concrete evidence of disease progression and the impact of any intervention.

It is beneficial to have a dedicated forum where members of the core care team can discuss each patient. The membership of this team will vary between institutions and settings but it is important to have a variety of disciplines present, rather than only nursing staff. The aim of the forum is to facilitate input from people involved in the patient's care who have different focuses and perspectives. A core care group consisting of a nurse, an occupational therapist or physiotherapist and a pastoral care worker, for example, can provide expertise and advice regarding the physical and functional, healthcare and spiritual aspects of the patient.

Each team member should have the added responsibility of extending core group involvement to important care team members who may be unable to meet regularly. For example a senior nurse may meet with the doctor involved in the patient's care to communicate information regarding the patient's condition, the effect of interventions and the input of the allied health team. Any changes in medication or management, and any factors that contraindicate proposed interventions, can then be taken back to the care team.

Specific referrals to allied health professionals such as dieticians, speech pathologists and psychologists should evolve organically from the discussions that occur in the team meeting. Any problem that arises should be discussed with a view to involving anyone who may be able to assist. For example, a speech pathologist is imperative for any patient with head and neck pathology, a history of stroke, chronic cough or reduced cognition. Their advice can help guide the care team with regard to feeding techniques, positioning and food textures.

The biggest barrier to optimising care is often not the inability of the care team to recognise the need; it is the unwillingness of the team to consider the possibility that someone 'from outside' can make a valuable contribution.

Any caring profession runs the risk of developing a feeling of 'ownership' of their patient. Doctors and nurses are well known for blurring the boundaries between professional care and invested involvement. The main barrier to the effective involvement of allied health professionals is often this subconscious reluctance to consider that anyone else could provide benefit to 'our' patient.

Consider the 'triangle of care' below and ask yourself which category of carer you fit into. Perhaps the category changes depending on which patient you're looking after, or what sort of day you've had?

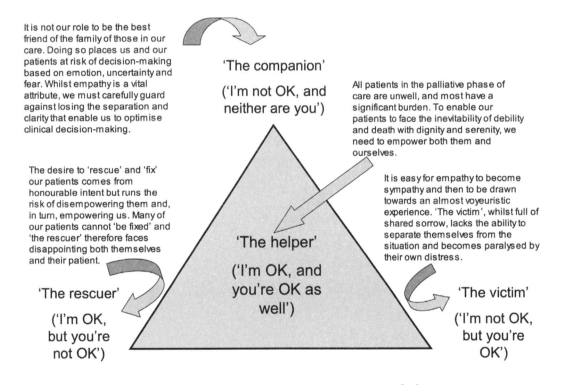

It is not our role to be the best friend of the family of those in our care. Doing so places us and our patients at risk of decision-making based on emotion, uncertainty and fear. Whilst empathy is a vital attribute, we must carefully guard against losing the separation and clarity that enable us to optimise clinical decision-making.

'The companion'

('I'm not OK, and neither are you')

All patients in the palliative phase of care are unwell, and most have a significant burden. To enable our patients to face the inevitability of debility and death with dignity and serenity, we need to empower both them and ourselves.

The desire to 'rescue' and 'fix' our patients comes from honourable intent but runs the risk of disempowering them and, in turn, empowering us. Many of our patients cannot 'be fixed' and 'the rescuer' therefore faces disappointing both themselves and their patient.

It is easy for empathy to become sympathy and then to be drawn towards an almost voyeuristic experience. 'The victim', whilst full of shared sorrow, lacks the ability to separate themselves from the situation and becomes paralysed by their own distress.

'The helper'

('I'm OK, and you're OK as well')

'The rescuer'

('I'm OK, but you're not OK')

'The victim'

('I'm not OK, but you're OK')

Figure 2.1 *Rescuer, companion, victim or helper?*

The risk of slipping into unhelpful care paradigms increases with patients that we like a lot, dislike a lot, or view as very similar to ourselves. We need to regularly analyse our own attitudes and motivation to ensure that we maintain a healthy and professional attitude in the face of often challenging situations. These issues are dealt with more fully in Chapter 14 but it is important to acknowledge that feeling like 'the only person able to rescue a patient' is one of the principal causes of failure to heed the advice of other health professionals.

However, situations can occur when the advice of one team member contradicts that of another, or when the aims of one do not fit easily with the aims of others. A situation where the dietician recommends increased intake of supplements due to poor protein levels or vitamin deficiency, and the nursing opinion is that the patient has no appetite and should not be burdened by increased intake, is such an example. Usually a simple discussion considering the holistic care of the patient can identify the appropriate approach.

In more difficult situations, it may only be possible to manage potential conflict by deferring to the most senior member of the group or to that member of the group who has the most responsibility. In many cases, this person will be the medical practitioner involved in the patient's care. It is also important to remember that the patient may have an opinion of their own, and they may be able to enlighten us as to the most beneficial course of action if we give them the time and opportunity to do so.

Palliative care versus the acute medical setting

Acute hospitals are busy, under-resourced and discharge-focused. They exist to diagnose and treat illness. It is therefore not surprising that many patients suitable for the palliative approach are managed very poorly in the acute hospital setting. By definition, palliative patients cannot be 'fixed'. Careful symptom control, with the aim of optimising quality of life, is not something at which over-stretched emergency departments or general medical wards of large hospitals excel.

Many health professionals, especially doctors, are trained always to aim for a cure. In the traditional medical model, the history and symptoms of the patient are synthesised and appropriate tests ordered, with the aim of treating and curing disease. For every symptom or sign, there are multiple possible tests. Physicians frequently feel a sense of failure when they are not able to achieve their aim of admission, diagnosis, treatment and resolution.

The palliative patient, who usually presents with chronic or progressive, previously documented and investigated illness, and who has no potential for cure or significant improvement challenges this medical paradigm. This dichotomy often leads to palliative patients having to undergo multiple tests and investigations. However, tests are only of value if the results can potentially lead to appropriate and beneficial intervention. Simple tests (such as mid-stream urine examinations) are not burdensome and can often result in the effective treatment of infection. Similarly, it is helpful to perform expensive imaging if there is a treatment that can be prescribed. But if the abnormality has been documented previously, and is known to be progressive (as in the case of malignancy), then re-imaging without a specific aim, for example palliative radiotherapy, is unhelpful. Before a palliative patient is sent for any invasive or burdensome investigation it is important for the care team to ask themselves not only what is likely to be found, but what treatment, if any, is possible and whether the findings are likely to change the treatment currently being prescribed.

Careful documentation and communication are vital in order to avoid burdensome and futile testing. Any elderly or unwell patient presenting at an Emergency Department can expect to receive basic blood tests, a chest x-ray and a urine test, but more extensive testing can often be avoided if clear information is given at the time of presentation regarding their diagnosis, prognosis, care aims and current treatments. It is unfair to blame medical staff for performing too many tests if they are not provided with thorough and contemporaneous information. Similarly, it is important to understand that, in some circumstances, there may be medico-legal reasons for performing certain investigations.

For many staff, the feeling that a ward patient they are caring for is being subjected to multiple inappropriate investigations is both frustrating and upsetting. In many cases, continuing investigation in the face of a well-documented and unequivocal palliative diagnosis represents a failure or reluctance on the part of the patient, the family or the doctor to accept the situation, or a failure to communicate the situation appropriately and effectively. Some patients will continue to demand rigorous testing, despite thorough explanation and evidence of its futility.

In some cases, it is the family members or carers who insist on repeated investigation. In this situation, it is important that several opportunities for discussion are documented and that the care team can demonstrate that they have discussed the issues involved and that the reasons for not ordering tests are also documented. A doctor is not obliged to order tests that they feel are contraindicated or futile, and the care team needs to present a consistent, firm and transparent front. If a patient wishes to pursue a more aggressive treatment plan, this should be documented and facilitated through referral for a second opinion from a suitably qualified doctor.

Continual investigation can often delay the ability of the patient, family and medical staff to move their own thinking from a curative to a palliative framework. It is understandably easier to focus on the most recent renal function results than to accept that the patient has end-stage renal failure and no longer wishes to be dialysed.

However, there are situations where patients are under-investigated and under-treated simply because they have been labelled as 'palliative'. Every presentation of every patient requires a separate, appropriate decision as to the best management strategy for the specific situation being encountered. For example, an 85-year-old man being managed with the palliative approach due to his dementia should not be denied proper investigations after a fall. Unfortunately, it still happens that a fractured neck of femur is discovered some days or weeks after a fall when a patient's altered behaviour is finally investigated. For *all* patients, careful documentation, thorough review and examination and patient-centred decision-making are the cornerstones in optimising outcome. Telephone calls, chart reviews and third-person observations do not constitute an examination of any patient and should not be accepted as such just because a patient is 'palliative'.

Chapter 3

Care of the elderly and dementia

In the past, many palliative care services were reluctant to get involved in care of the elderly. Being old and having dementia was regarded as a condition that was 'normal' and was not thought to require the involvement of specialist palliative care. For the most part, this is true. However, many of the management strategies utilised in palliative care can be easily and effectively used in the context of care for the elderly.

The general population continues to age, and geriatric medicine is now a major growth industry around the world. For instance, according to the US government 'Administration on Aging' website in 2000 people over the age of 65 represented 12.9% of the American population, but by 2030 it is estimated that they will account for at least 19%.

Unfortunately, geriatric patients, along with psychiatric and palliative care patients, still suffer discrimination in most societies. The breakdown of the nuclear family, and the reluctance and inability of younger family members to care for the elderly, mean that Western society is facing a pandemic of aging. Acute medicine has done all it can for many of these patients, and their health is deteriorating in a predictable and non-dramatic fashion. The symptom complexes that impact most on their quality of life can frequently be managed in the community, and transfer to the acute setting can often be avoided.

When considering the care needs of elderly patients, it is helpful to distinguish burdens that are attributable to specific medical conditions, for example, dyspnoea due to obstructive airways disease, from burdens due to old age, such as degenerative bone disease, memory impairment and decreased visual acuity and from issues such as spiritual or psychiatric morbidity. People manage the challenges of aging in a variety of ways, ranging from dignified acceptance and gratitude for longevity to bitter resentment and anger at the ravages of time. An individual's attitude can have a huge impact on their quality of life, and it is important for staff to be aware of what constitutes normal aging so that patients in their care can be encouraged and supported.

Normal aging

Every organ and system ages differently in each individual. The following points summarise the changes that are part of normal aging:

- **Vision**: It is usual for the lens of the eye to stiffen in the forties or fifties and lead to a need for reading glasses. Peripheral vision reduces, colour clarity is diminished and glare becomes more of a problem.

- **Hearing**: After the mid-fifties, it is usual for hearing acuity to diminish, especially at higher frequencies. If there is background noise, distinguishing voices becomes more difficult.

- **Taste and smell**: Overall taste sensitivity declines and saliva production may be reduced, leading to a dry mouth. The olfactory senses also decline with age.

- **Bone**: By mid-life, bone mineral loss is occurring faster than bone replacement. This change is accelerated in post-menopausal women and by coffee drinking and cigarette smoking. Height is lost through a combination of postural change and joint/disc compression. Joints suffer increasingly from 'wear and tear', with progressive aching and stiffness.

- **Muscle and fat**: Fat deposition increases until middle age, stabilises and then declines. Fat shifts from being predominantly subcutaneous to being predominantly central. Muscle mass declines, and this results in slowing of the metabolism.

- **Skin**: Skin loses elasticity and becomes thinner. The capacity to heal is reduced, and nail and hair growth also slows.

- **Urinary system**: The kidneys shrink and become less efficient and the bladder becomes less able to distend which leads to the need for more frequent urination.

- **Sexual function**: Both men and women produce fewer sex hormones. Menopausal women cease ovulation and vaginal lubrication declines. Male sperm production falls and sexual response time increases.

- **Brain**: The size, blood flow and neuronal network of the brain start to decrease somewhere around the age of 40. New networks and adaptations can still occur but, by the seventh decade, reduced short-term memory and slower recall of specific pieces of information are common. As we age, we rely increasingly on concrete pre-established patterns to manage information. The rapid assimilation of new information becomes more difficult and reflexes are slowed.

- **Heart**: The heart muscle thickens with age, and maximum heart rates decline.
- **Lungs**: Lung tissue gradually loses elasticity, and the muscles of the rib cage shrink. The lungs' vital capacity for both inspiration and expiration decreases, and the effectiveness of gaseous exchange declines.
- **Arteries**: The arteries stiffen with age, and atherosclerotic accumulation can further reduce blood flow.
- **Metabolic change**: The slowing of all body systems results in slower metabolism of medications, slower excretion rates and the potential for accumulation. There is a reduced energy requirement and increased fatigue.

Dementia

Dementia is not a diagnosis in itself. There are many different causes of dementia. It is generally defined as a decline in intellectual functioning, with associated problems of memory, reasoning and thinking. Dementia must be differentiated from the more acute and fluctuating changes caused by delirium. Dementia is very rare in younger age groups, and more common in people older than 70.

The most common types are Alzheimer's type dementia and vascular dementia. Dementia can also be associated with Parkinson's disease. There are many other causes, which may or may not be amenable to treatment, including certain vitamin deficiencies, acquired immune deficiency syndrome (AIDS), progressive supranuclear palsy, Huntington's disease and Wilson's disease. There are also cases of rapidly progressive dementia due to relatively rare conditions such as Creutzfeldt-Jakob disease (CJD). Due to the wide variety of causes, and the fact that some types of dementia can be slowed and occasionally even reversed by treatment, accurate diagnosis by a qualified doctor (preferably a geriatrician) is vital.

Alzheimer's disease

Alzheimer's disease is a neurodegenerative form of dementia that is common in the elderly and used to be called 'senile dementia'. It is characterised by neuronal loss and the development of abnormal aggregates of protein, resulting in tangles and plaques in the brain. The cause is unknown.

Most patients are brought to medical attention because of progressive impairment of memory (particularly short-term memory). Writing and other fine motor skills may become more difficult, and patients often become unable to plan and execute complex multi-stage tasks. Later in the disease, long-term memory may be affected, and behavioural, language and psychiatric problems become more common. The disease progresses relentlessly until patients lose the ability to manage activities of daily living and become reliant on care. Mobility and speech are often lost in the advanced stage of the disease and patients become bed-bound and physically wasted and exhausted.

Alzheimer's disease is a terminal illness but many patients live well with the disease for years. The rate of its progression varies. Death usually occurs due to complications caused by the disease, such as pneumonia.

Vascular and multi-infarct dementia

After Alzheimer's disease, the most common form of dementia in the elderly is vascular dementia, or dementia caused by compromised blood flow to the brain. Multi-infarct dementia is one type of vascular dementia. Clinically, it is often impossible to distinguish one type of vascular dementia from another. All vascular dementias are the result of cerebrovascular disease and many patients present after suffering a stroke.

A stroke can be either haemorrhagic (caused by bleeding) or ischaemic (caused by a clot that restricts the blood supply). In the majority of patients, a pervasive pattern of small vessel disease in the brain causes a step-wise deterioration in cognitive function. Although vascular dementia is not curable, the risk factors for it – which include high blood pressure, diabetes and cigarette smoking – can be modified.

End-stage dementia

Progressive dementia is a terminal diagnosis but most families and many healthcare professionals do not recognise this. Patients with end-stage dementia have lost the ability to manage their own activities of daily living and are dependent on nursing care. In most cases, language has been lost, or reduced to single words, and the agitation that may have been a feature earlier in the disease has usually subsided. These patients are often bed-bound and frail, with contractures of some or all limbs and minimal intake of food and fluid.

Patients at this stage of dementia are unable to describe their symptoms so behavioural pain scales and visual scales, with an emphasis on facial expression, are used. The palliative approach, which emphasises comfort and dignity, is the optimal care paradigm at this point. Patients with end-stage dementia are unable to move at will and may develop widespread 'bed-ache'. But the simple provision of regular analgesia is often overlooked – because 'he/she never complains' and staff forget that the patient is unable to say anything at all. Often, the initial use of liquid paracetamol, followed by a topical agent (in patch form) such as buprenorphine or fentanyl, begun at a low dose and titrated gradually based on need, is the single most beneficial intervention. The provision of as-needed analgesia, such as liquid morphine prior to turning, and careful attention to issues such as oral hygiene and eye care can provide great relief of distress.

Chapter 4
Old age

To the 'normal' symptoms of aging, we need to add symptoms related to the common diseases of old age, particularly the joint pain and stiffness of osteoarthritis, and the symptoms related to the 'lifestyle diseases' that are so prevalent in Western society. Obesity and type 2 diabetes involve many symptoms, including joint pain, fatigue and sleep disturbance. By the time we reach 80, few of us are likely to escape a diagnosis of one or more of a plethora of diseases, such as ischaemic heart disease, cerebrovascular disease, obstructive airways disease, depression, anxiety, chronic degenerative back pain, visual impairment or hearing loss. According to the website of Arthritis NSW, one of the leading arthritis networks in Australia, around 18% of the Australian population suffer from arthritis and it accounts for approximately 75% of expenditure on care for the elderly. When we add the morbidity related to other, more specific diagnoses, it is clear that the average resident in an elderly care facility is likely to have a significant symptom burden.

However, for many of these symptoms, there are simple and effective interventions that can be instituted as part of a supportive care package. For example, the addition of regular paracetamol, a soft diet, pressure care, a low-dose anti-depressant and appropriate mild laxatives (aperients) may be all that is required to significantly improve the quality of life for an elderly patient. Conscientious multidisciplinary assessment is vital in order to identify the need for such interventions.

The following three case studies of 'typical' elderly patients highlight the way in which the palliative approach can be used to enhance quality of life. Each of the following patients and/or their families had made the decision to decline resuscitation or transfer to an acute facility.

Mrs B. D. (Beryl)

Beryl was an 84-year-old woman with moderate dementia living in a care home for the elderly. Beryl had a medical history that included a cerebro-vascular accident (CVA) or stroke five years earlier, which had resulted in some residual left-sided weakness, diabetes, peripheral vascular disease, ischaemic heart disease with occasional angina pain but no infarction (heart attack), osteoarthritis and a hysterectomy. Over the last year, her function had steadily declined with worsening joint pain, increased shortness of breath, episodic nausea and worsening symptoms of memory loss, confusion and agitation.

Beryl was reviewed systematically by the nurse responsible for her care, her general practitioner (GP) and an occupational therapist. When all the information was reviewed, the following picture emerged :

- Generalised joint aches and pains, maximal in the hips and back. Known osteoporosis and osteoarthritis but pain is now impacting on mobility and sleep.
- Fearful when mobilising due to recent fall.
- Increased difficulty managing multiple oral medications. Frequent episodes of medications being missed due to nausea and non-compliance.
- No vomiting but oral intake has declined over the last six months.
- Nausea, particularly after taking morning and evening medications.
- Gradual weight loss and constipation with bowel movements every three or four days.
- Episodic confusion and agitation, which is worse at night and with changes in routine.
- Vaginal thrush and excoriation evident on examination.

Beryl's case was discussed by the care team and her medications were reviewed. Her medication list included three blood pressure tablets, an oral hypoglycaemic (a medication for diabetes), a lipid-lowering drug, aspirin, benzodiazepine (a sedative) at night and as-needed paracetamol and diazepam.

The team requested blood pressure (BP) and blood sugar (BSL) measurements over a few days and subsequently:

- Lipid-lowering medication and two anti-hypertensives were ceased. *Nausea and unsteadiness improved.*
- Beryl was started on regular paracetamol liquid four times a day. *Hip and back pain improved.*
- She was treated with oral fluconazole. *Thrush and excoriation resolved.*

- Her BSL was repeatedly noted to be high and she was changed to slow-release insulin at night. *Incidence of urinary tract infection (UTI) and fungal and yeast infections declined.*

- Regular laxatives were instituted. *Constipation improved.*

- Beryl was enrolled in a fall prevention programme but she was non-compliant. She was given a walking frame and a wheelchair for outings.

- A nightlight was provided and benzodiazepines gradually reduced and then ceased.

Beryl's mobility remained poor, and episodes of confusion and agitation continued (albeit much less frequently). Constipation, nausea and complaints of pain became very infrequent. A plan was documented that ensured monitoring of Beryl's compliance with oral paracetamol and suggested topical buprenorphine patches if compliance worsened and pain was still an issue. A referral to a psychogeriatrician was arranged to facilitate optimal prescribing for agitation and the collection of high-quality information to form the basis of a behavioural review. The GP documented the option of low-dose antipsychotic medication for agitation at night and gave clear guidelines for its use.

This case illustrates the fact that, for many elderly patients, simple measures can be very effective. Medication review with the aim of minimising tablet intake should be approached diligently, with the question being not so much 'which medication can we cease?' as 'why shouldn't we cease this medication?' For many elderly patients, long-term prevention (such as reducing the risk of stroke by using cholesterol-lowering agents) is irrelevant and the burden, including nausea, is significant. Simple adjustments – such as changing analgesics to topical creams or patches, changing anti-emetics and anti-depressants to dispersible tablets or wafers and considering sustained-release insulin instead of multiple oral hypoglycaemics – can be very beneficial. Careful physical examination is paramount and there is no excuse for any clinician to ignore issues such as rectal pain, vaginal discharge or genital pain, based on a patient's age and a misguided concern about causing embarrassment.

Miss I. M. (Ivy)

Ivy was a 92-year-old woman with end-stage dementia. She had been treated with combined chemo-radiation for colon cancer 18 years earlier and had persistent and very frequent diarrhoea. Ivy was bed-bound and had been non-verbal for over a year. She was cachexic and her oral intake was poor. She had contractures of most joints. Most of Ivy's medications had been stopped a month earlier when it was presumed she was dying.

Ivy was reviewed by the nurse and volunteer who looked after her, a physiotherapist and the local doctor. They phoned her niece, who visited weekly and had expressed concern about Ivy's condition several times. The following facts were noted:

- She often moaned on turning and the staff felt she had pain on movement.

- Pain when being fed and when the light was switched on in her room.

- Pressure area on the medial aspect of both heels, on the sacrum and helix (rim) of her left ear.

- On further examination, oral thrush, xerostomia and a corneal ulcer due to dryness were noted.

- Abdominal examination revealed a palpable mass.

Ivy's niece was invited to meet the care team and the situation was reviewed. After discussion, the decision was made not to further investigate the abdominal finding, and a presumptive diagnosis of malignancy was made.

- Ivy was started on a fentanyl patch. *Comfort improved rapidly.*

- Physiotherapy and occupational therapy review resulted in a pressure-care mattress and improved positioning. *Although the pressure areas did not resolve, there was no further deterioration and comfort improved.*

- Anti-fungal drops and regular saliva substitute were commenced. *Oral intake improved slightly and comfort improved.*

- After phone advice from an ophthalmologist, specific eye drops were commenced and subsequently replaced with regular lubricant drops. *Photophobia resolved.*

- Several medications were trialled for diarrhoea but they were limited by poor oral intake and nausea. Careful hygiene and barrier creams improved local skin integrity.

Ivy died four weeks later. The staff caring for her felt that she had been very comfortable and her niece contacted the nursing home to thank them for the care they had given her aunt.

Ivy's case illustrates the importance of effective analgesia in patients with dementia who may be unable to tolerate regular oral analgesics and who have a limited ability to express their pain. Feedback from the staff who care for the patient on a day-to-day basis and the views of close family or friends are vital in order to assess pain properly in this patient group. For example, lesions of the mouth and eyes are painful and distressing and are often caused by dryness. They can be prevented by the simple provision of artificial tears and saliva. Many doctors may be unfamiliar with treating specific eye complaints but it is important to seek advice and assistance if needed.

Most specialists are happy to give advice over the phone and the biggest barrier is often the care team's unwillingness to ask for help. For any patient with pressure sores or decreased mobility, it is always beneficial to organise a review by an occupational therapist and physiotherapist as quickly as possible. In the final stages of dementia, pain relief is the paramount concern and families are finely tuned to the discomfort of their loved one. Good nursing care, appropriate analgesia and careful explanation will usually make the inability to resolve an issue like diarrhoea inconsequential in the terminal phase.

Mr A.S. (Arthur)

Arthur was a 78-year-old man with advanced dementia and a history of psychotic features. He was admitted to a dementia-specific unit after being cared for by his wife at home for many years, when his behaviour became more aggressive. He had a history of significant alcohol abuse in the past, although he had not had any alcohol for several years. His medical history included osteoarthritis, known ischaemic heart disease, and chronic obstructive pulmonary disease due to smoking and asthma. He was still physically quite able and mobilised unaided. His confusion could be quite severe overnight and he had lashed out at staff.

Arthur's case was reviewed by the registered nurse in charge of the unit, one of the enrolled nurses familiar with Arthur's overnight care and an occupational therapist.

- After discussion it was clear that the staff were fed up with Arthur, and that his behaviour, especially overnight, had been causing problems for some time. The staff felt that none of their concerns regarding the situation had been listened to or acted upon.
- Arthur was often non-compliant with inhaled medications.
- Over the three weeks before the review, in addition to his regular nightly dose of 20mg of temazepam (a sedative), he had been given an olanzepine wafer (an atypical anti-psychotic medication used for behavioural disturbance and sedation) on most nights.
- Restraints had been used an average of three nights a week.

The staff realised that they did not have the expertise needed to manage the complexities of Arthur's case without assistance. The GP, who had been contacted many times regarding Arthur's case during previous months, declined to meet the care team. The decision was made to transfer Arthur's care to another GP in the same practice.

A psychologist's review was requested and, although there was a significant delay of three weeks before all members of the group had reviewed Arthur and could meet, the resulting information was very helpful.

- After discussions with his family, it was revealed that Arthur had been a prisoner of war and had slept with the light on for many years.

- His oxygen saturations were very variable overnight and, although it was impossible to perform formal sleep studies, he seemed to have prolonged periods of apnoea.

- He had widespread joint pain on palpation.

- A simple dip-stick urine test revealed a urinary tract infection.

- He was constipated.

Arthur was commenced on regular paracetamol and laxatives. He refused oral antibiotics and was given a single, immediate, intramuscular injection (stat IM) antibiotic dose. Overnight, non-invasive ventilation support (BiPap) was tried but, as expected, Arthur could not tolerate the machine and the noise worsened his anxiety and agitation. He was commenced on overnight oxygen via nasal prongs and, although he continued to have episodes of non-compliance, his sleep pattern improved. The psychologist sought advice from a psychiatrist, who reviewed Arthur and he was commenced on regular mood-stabilising medications. Benzodiazepines (sedative drugs such as diazepam and temazepam) were gradually reduced. Arthur was commenced on an oral bronchodilator (anti-asthma medication) due to continued issues with inhaled medications. His routine was regularised as much as possible and he was allowed to sleep with the light on.

Arthur's care remained challenging but the interventions resulted in a significant improvement in his overall quality of life. The number of aggressive outbursts reduced and the use of restraints became unnecessary. On review, the principal benefit of the multidisciplinary team process was deemed to be that staff caring for Arthur felt that their concerns had been listened to and acted upon. As a result, their attitude to him improved.

Old age is incurable. The symptom burdens endured by elderly patients can be significant but much can be done to improve their comfort and quality of life. Many of the interventions outlined above are relatively simple. The most important step is to recognise that even very small improvements can benefit not only the patient, but also the family and the staff.

Chapter 5
Death and dying

Everything that lives must die – and 100% of people will die. For something so common, our society copes with death very badly! There are obviously many factors to consider when we try to understand contemporary attitudes to death and dying in affluent, industrialised countries. Attitudes to death (which should not be confused with grief, which is a universal human emotion) are often very different in developing countries. Unfortunately, an exploration of death and dying in traditional and tribal cultures is beyond the scope of this book (Groves & Klauser 2005). However, it is impossible to overstate the importance of cultural sensitivity when dealing with these issues. Local community or church leaders can provide invaluable guidance on managing the terminal phase and death of patients from particular religious or cultural groups.

Changing attitudes to death

When we look back at the mummification rituals and elaborate tombs of ancient Egypt, or the mourning fashions and deathbed photography of the Victorians, we refer to them as being 'obsessed with death'. However, in centuries to come, I am sure our own period of civilisation will be considered 'death-avoiding'. As a society, we are intellectually aware of the inevitability of death but we studiously avoid the subject throughout our lives. It is only discussed when we are confronted by our own mortality or that of someone we care about. The generation of people who grew up in households that routinely cared for relatives dying at home are now growing old themselves. Close extended family is becoming a rarity and nuclear families are often fractured. Dying at home is relatively uncommon outside the group of people who die suddenly, often from myocardial infarction.

Governments would like to encourage dying at home, as many people express a desire to die in the place they are most familiar with and the cost savings are significant. However, when the situation actually presents itself, many patients who had expressed a desire to die at home grow fearful and recognise the value of the security they feel when surrounded by trained staff. Care of the dying requires 24-hour continuous effort and many families are simply unable to manage issues such as bowel care, washing and turning, let alone symptoms such as vomiting, diarrhoea, pain and breathlessness. Large resources are being devoted to improving the rates for dying at home but it is still much more usual for death to occur in an institution such as a nursing home or hospital.

Death is no longer part of the continuum of life as it was in the days when viewing the deceased, often in the parlour or hall, was the usual prelude to the wake. The days when the majority of families lost children during childbirth or in the first few years of life, and when infectious diseases such as tuberculosis and smallpox carried a high chance of mortality, have long gone. As a result, our communal understanding is that death is something that occurs, usually in a hospital bed, when the fight to keep a person alive has been lost.

Accepting death

Our group consciousness accepts the great advances of modern medicine and somehow forgets the human frailty that may have been supported by a cocktail of anti-hypertensives (for blood pressure), hypoglycaemics (for diabetes), beta-blockers (for heart failure) and a pacemaker for years. Healthcare professionals often forget that, for many people, the death of even elderly and unwell loved ones is a shock. The shock is even more profound when people die at a younger age. Many people find it difficult to accept the concept of diseases that cannot be cured or at least have their effects mitigated.

Contemporary Western society is largely based on the concepts of autonomy and control. We place a great deal of trust in justice, cause and effect, and in the power of science and money to solve our health problems. For example, when we are confronted with a fulminant malignancy in a young person that has not responded to any of the available treatments, we demand newer and better treatments, more medications, a second opinion, someone to blame. It is natural, of course, to strive to do all that we can. But losing sight of the fundamental truth that 'all that lives must die' places an intolerable burden not only on the patient and family, but also on the healthcare staff. Some patients feel this burden so acutely that they feel guilty about dying, as though they have somehow given up a noble fight.

For some people, religious faith enables them to accept the concept of death with more serenity, but it would be a mistake to conclude that faith eases the acceptance of death for all those who hold it. Very few healthcare workers who routinely care for dying people have not listened to the questions of religious people who cannot understand why their faith is not being rewarded. Just as our education teaches us the laws of cause and effect, we often assume that religious observance will somehow result in protection from terminal illness and death. Many people in this situation feel abandoned and let down by their religion, and believe they are being punished by God. These spiritual battles largely result from the fundamental fear we have of death and dying.

To die means to leave behind everything we know and to be separated forever from our loved ones. It's natural to grieve about this separation from people we care about. However, holding in our hearts a deep fear of death itself is based on our ignorance of the process of death and of what, if anything, happens after death. The latter question is, of course, one of life's great mysteries but education can help patients and families dispel some of the fears and misconception surrounding the dying process.

Talking about death

The first hurdle to overcome is the fact that we are taught from a young age that death is not something that is readily discussed. The majority of people with advanced and incurable illness are well aware of the inevitability of death, but it is often not openly talked about, even amongst close family and friends.

When healthcare professionals facilitate the discussion, however, the resulting opportunity can be very beneficial. The fundamental skills needed to discuss death with a patient are not complex and the task, whilst initially confronting, becomes easier with familiarity. Honest and simple language, empathy and compassion and an awareness of non-verbal cues are the best starting points.

There are many different ways to initiate a conversation about dying, and much will depend on the particular patient and the environment. The initial approach is usually the most difficult part. Starting the conversation with a question can often make things easier:

'Leanne, you seem much weaker than yesterday. Things seem to be changing every day. I think that time is short. What do you think?'

'Many people we look after are frightened about what actually happens when people die. Is there anything that's been worrying you or that you are scared about?'

'Tom, looking at Alice now, I think that she might die quite soon. Have you been thinking that as well?'

'You seem completely worn out. Sometimes people just feel so tired that they want to go to sleep and not wake up. Is that how you're feeling?'

'Often as people get closer to death, their breathing becomes more irregular. Have you noticed that with Arthur?'

'It's very difficult to predict when someone will die, but Margaret's condition has changed a lot since this morning. Do you feel that she will die soon?'

Many patients and their family members have deep fears regarding the dying process and they are often too embarrassed to ask questions without being prompted. It is important to give all patients and carers the opportunity to reveal these fears. However, it may sometimes be more beneficial to address any obvious concern directly, without relying on the ability of the patient or family member to express their concerns verbally. The aim is to normalise the concern, and to educate and reassure. The fear of dying of dehydration, suffocation or in severe pain is common, and careful explanation of the dying process (see Chapter 10) can alleviate their distress and anxiety:

'Bill, lots of people with lung cancer, who are short of breath, worry that they'll suffocate. Have you had those sorts of worries? What actually happens is that, as dying gets closer, the body relaxes and breathing is not so difficult. We can give you medication to reduce the feeling of being short of breath and keep you comfortable.'

'Lots of people ask me what happens when people die. It's not something that we talk about much, is it? Do you have any questions about what might happen as Rose gets closer to dying?'

In fact, for the majority of people, death occurs peacefully whilst in a coma state, and it can be very comforting to explain this. Some patients and their families ask quite detailed questions regarding the process of the certification of death and what will happen to the body immediately following death. Careful discussion of the procedures (including checking for the absence of pulse, heart activity and breathing, and ascertaining that the pupils no longer react to light and that there is no response to physical stimuli) can alleviate fears that death will somehow be 'misdiagnosed'. Portraying death as an expected sequel to the disease processes that have led to the palliative phase of care, rather than an unexpected or acute event, can greatly ameliorate these fears.

Helping patients and families to develop an understanding and acceptance of dying is a vital part of palliative management. It should also be seen as an important intervention that can reduce the instance of pathological grieving (see Chapter 13). Some people have problems relating to the death of a loved one that stem from their own difficulties with the concept of death and dying, and these individuals may need referral to a psychologist or psychiatrist. Caring for a patient in the palliative phase should be seen as a unique opportunity to provide education and support that can positively affect the attitudes of several generations and, through them, serve as a conduit of information into the wider community.

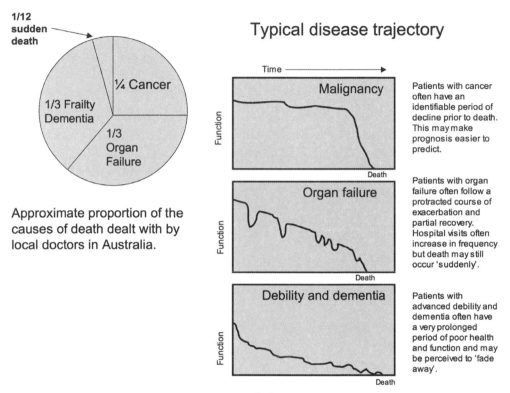

Approximate proportion of the causes of death dealt with by local doctors in Australia.

Figure 5.1 *Typical disease trajectory*

Chapter 6
Malignancy

It is difficult to over-estimate the impact that a diagnosis of 'cancer' has on a patient and their loved ones. Cancer is defined by the uncontrolled division of abnormal cells, the ability to invade normal tissue and often by the ability to spread (metastasise) to remote areas of the body via the bloodstream or lymphatic system.

However, there are actually more than 100 different types of cancer. Cancers are often named after the area where they originate – for example 'breast cancer' and 'bowel cancer'. Cancer that metastasises to another area retains the structure of the tissue where it originated. Therefore breast cancer that has spread to the brain is referred to as 'breast cancer with brain metastases'.

In addition to this anatomical division, we divide cancer into groups based on broader origin. Carcinoma is derived from skin or the linings or coverings of organs (for example, squamous cell carcinoma of the skin and adenocarcinoma of the bowel). Sarcomas develop in bone, cartilage, fat, blood vessels, muscles and other supportive and connective tissues. Leukaemia is a cancer of blood-producing tissues, while lymphoma/myeloma are cancers of the immune system.

Cancer is further described based on its appearance under the microscope, and its aggressiveness and degree of deviation from normal tissue. It is important to remember that, in many cases, there are degrees of deviation from normal, and the change from 'completely normal' to 'frankly malignant' may follow a continuum. The best-known example of this is cervical smear results, in which cells that are slightly abnormal often normalise but occasionally progress towards more cancerous change. If the cells are localised, and can be completely removed by surgery or radiotherapy, the cancer may be curable. Prognosis is determined by many complex factors, including the specific type and grade of the cancer, the location and the degree of spread, as well as the physical condition of the patient and their response to treatment.

For the purposes of this book we will use simple anatomical names and will not cover grading systems or rarer variations. There are several well-established factors that are known to cause cancer (for example, cigarette smoke and the human papilloma virus) but in many cases the aetiology is complex. For this reason, we refer to 'risk factors'. Some cancers are known to have a genetic predisposition but in most cases there are multiple risk factors for any given type of cancer, and many cases arise without obvious cause.

Tiredness, weakness, weight loss and reduction in appetite are pervasive symptoms in most types of cancer. Cancer cells cause changes in the body's fluid chemistry and are voracious consumers of energy. Cancers vary enormously in their cell type, location, behaviour and aggressiveness. Patients with the same diagnosis may therefore experience completely different patterns of disease progression and treatment response. Some patients can appear quite well with a large volume of cancer, whereas others may appear close to death with what appears to be a very small volume of disease.

This chapter gives some general information about common cancers but is not intended to provide anything other than a brief overview and readers are encouraged to refer to specialist texts (Bruera & Yennurajalingam 2012, Caraceni, Hanks, *et al.* 2012, Twycross, Wilcock, *et al.* 2009).

Some common malignancies

Brain tumours

'Brain tumour' is a collective term used to describe a variety of solid growths that occur in the brain. They occur in both adults and children. Tumours from other areas may metastasise to the brain and these are referred to as 'secondary' or 'metastatic' brain tumours. But tumours that originate in the brain rarely metastasise to other areas.

The concept of 'benign' and 'malignant' is not as straightforward when considering brain tumours as it is with other tumours – simply because of the anatomy involved. The brain is a vulnerable vital organ, protected by the rigid bones of the skull. Any space-occupying lesion, be it technically benign or malignant, has the potential to cause death by compressing normal brain tissue.

Malignant cerebral tumours can progress slowly or rapidly, and a 'low-grade' tumour can rapidly turn into a 'high-grade' one. Tumours are usually found after a patient experiences headache, nausea, personality change, seizures or some other neurological change such as clumsiness and weakness. Tumour bulk can be removed by surgery but, in the majority of cases, the tumour has sent out thread-like projections into the surrounding brain tissue, and cancer cells remain and the disease recurs. Many brain tumours are also 'multi-focal', which makes surgery impossible due to the amount of normal brain tissue that would be damaged. Radiotherapy can be employed to treat a local area (with the aim of preventing, or slowing recurrence) or to treat the whole brain.

Steroid medications can be used to reduce the swelling associated with the tumour. The symptoms from brain tumours are often due to pressure effects, which can give patients headaches, nausea and seizures in advanced disease. Some patients may experience increasing agitation, which may require specialist intervention and sedation. Drowsiness followed by coma is the most frequent terminal change in this patient group. Surgery and steroid medications can have impressive effects in many patients. This may lead families to struggle with terminal deterioration because previous downturns have perhaps responded to medication and the patient appears physically well, often without the wasting and weight loss that accompany many other cancers.

Breast cancer

Breast cancer is a complex group of diseases that represents the most common cause of cancer-related deaths in women. Men can also get breast cancer. Multiple risk factors (including age, oestrogen exposure and radiation) have been identified, and approximately 5% of breast cancer is genetically linked. Breast cancer can vary from a slow-growing, relatively indolent disease that women live with for decades to a rapidly progressive and aggressive disease that can cause death in young women despite optimised treatment.

A breast mass is a frequent presenting symptom but many women have metastatic disease at diagnosis. The most common sites for metastatic spread are skin, bone, liver, lung and brain. Treatment options include surgery and radiotherapy, and a variety of hormonal and chemotherapy options based on specific cancer characteristics. Some women experience an added psychiatric burden because of the disfiguring results of surgery and the impact of the surgery on their psychosexual function.

In the palliative stage of care, the main issues related to breast cancer are local skin infiltration, which can lead to painful, bleeding and odorous wounds; the management of painful swelling of the arm (lymphoedema), which can result from surgery and radiation; and the management of symptoms related to metastatic disease, particularly bone pain.

Colon cancer

Colon cancer is 'bowel cancer' occurring in the large intestine but any area of the gastrointestinal tract can be affected by malignancy. Colorectal cancer is a common type of cancer in Western society and risk factors include diet, inflammatory bowel disease and genetic predisposition. The symptoms of bowel cancer depend on its location but may include abdominal pain, diarrhoea, constipation, severe weight loss, bleeding from the bowel and intestinal blockage.

Surgery remains a mainstay of treatment and is augmented by chemotherapy and radiotherapy as required. The initial surgical procedures may be extensive and involve the formation of a stoma and the subsequent use of external stoma bags to manage faecal waste. The prognosis of bowel cancer is related to the size of the tumour, its location and its degree of spread. Some patients with local disease that has been completely removed may simply require regular follow-up, whereas others may have advanced disease that spreads to the liver and lung. Problems with managing diet, constipation and/or recurrent diarrhoea and intestinal obstruction (with resulting abdominal pain and vomiting) are issues in these patients.

Gynaecological cancer

Cancer of the cervix, ovaries and other parts of the genital tract make up around 20% of cancers in women in developed countries. Cervical cancer is often detected by routine PAP (cervical smear) screening but ovarian cancer may present very late. Symptoms of cervical cancer include bleeding, painful intercourse and pelvic pain, and ovarian cancer may present with abdominal pain, bloating or bowel changes. Cancer of the lining of the uterus may present with vaginal bleeding.

The principal risk factor for cervical cancer is human papilloma virus (HPV) but smoking is also implicated. In early disease, localised procedures can remove the affected area of the cervix but more advanced disease may require total hysterectomy, extensive pelvic surgery and radiation treatment. Metastatic disease is treated with chemotherapy but it is an aggressive cancer and responds poorly. The issues particularly related to patients with cervical cancer include problems with sexual function and self-esteem, pelvic pain and the fact that, like breast cancer, it can affect young women during their child-bearing years.

Ovarian cancer tends to be diagnosed in women in their fifties or older but it often presents late and has a poor prognosis for this reason. Ovarian cancer can be treated with surgery, radiation, chemotherapy or a combination of modalities. This cancer may spread by 'seeding' into the abdominal cavity and patients may experience abdominal pain, bloating and have a high risk of bowel obstruction, resulting in abdominal pain, vomiting, distension and inability to tolerate oral intake.

Head and neck cancers

The head and neck cancers are a diverse group of cancers that have in common the fact that they affect a part of the body with which we confront the world. The associated psychosocial impact of these cancers can therefore be severe. Alcohol consumption and cigarette smoking are the biggest risk factors. Squamous cell carcinoma arising from the skin and mucosal lining is the most frequent type but other structures (such as the larynx, the salivary glands and the palate) can also be involved.

Extensive and complex surgery may be required, and many patients also undergo combined radiotherapy and chemotherapy. Treatment can result in scarring, fibrosis and impaired ability to swallow. Patients undergoing high-dose radiotherapy may need inpatient care, due to difficult pain management (requiring high-dose opioid medications), dehydration and feeding issues. Some patients need to rely on nasogastric feeding in the short term, and PEG (a feeding tube inserted through the skin into the stomach or intestine) feeding in the long term.

Leukaemia

Leukaemia (or 'blood cancer') can be acute or chronic, and can affect several different types of white blood cells. Abnormal cells proliferate and the normal infection-fighting action of white blood cells is lost. Leukaemia can affect both adults and children and in some cases an indolent chronic form can change into a rapidly progressive acute form of the disease. There are several syndromes that are termed 'myelodysplastic'. These syndromes are often considered to be 'pre-leukaemia' states and may transform into acute leukaemia. However, some patients live comfortably with an altered blood picture for many years.

Treatment for leukaemia consists of aggressive chemotherapy and may include transfusions and bone marrow or stem cell transplants. Many patients experience a pattern of disease remission and relapse, with each subsequent remission becoming shorter. The prognosis for childhood leukaemia is significantly better than the prognosis for adults.

Many patients decide to adopt a palliative approach to care when they consider the burden of repeated transfusions. Earlier in the disease phase, patients often benefit from transfusion for many weeks and gain a good quality of life but, as the disease progresses, the benefit can become negligible. Palliative patients frequently experience symptoms related to the fact that their normal blood cells have been replaced by abnormal cells. They are therefore profoundly anaemic and lose the ability to clot. They may also experience fatigue, shortness of breath, bone pains and bleeding problems. Because the immune system is so severely compromised by leukaemia, death can occur very rapidly due to infection.

Lung cancer

There are several different types of lung cancer and together they account for around one-third of all cancer deaths. The best-known risk factors for lung cancer are cigarette smoking and asbestos exposure, but people can get lung cancer without exposure to either of these.

Many lung cancer patients who have been, or still are, cigarette smokers are aware that some members of the community feel that 'they deserve it' in some way, due to their smoking. These patients may also feel a personal sense of guilt about smoking. The most common symptoms of lung cancer are coughing, shortness of breath, chest pain and the coughing up of blood or blood-stained sputum. Treatment depends on the cell types involved, with small cell type lung cancers responding better to chemotherapy than large cell types. Surgery and radiotherapy (or combined treatments) are used, depending on the extent and location of the disease.

Lung cancer often spreads to bone, liver and brain and many patients develop 'pleural effusion' – fluid collecting around the lung that compresses normal lung tissue and results in shortness of breath and chest pain. Shortness of breath (with associated anxiety) is probably the most troublesome symptom in lung cancer patients. Most people have a deep-rooted anxiety about suffocation, and much of the care for patients with lung cancer in the terminal phase is focused on this symptom. In addition to breathlessness, many patients experience a variety of other symptoms associated with cancer including weight loss, fatigue, weakness and nausea.

Lymphoma

The lymphomas are a large and very diverse group of cancers of the immune system. There are many different types, which are distinguished according to their cellular origin. The most common symptoms at presentation are painless swellings of the lymph nodes. Many patients also experience itching, night sweats, fever and weight loss. On scanning, patients may have very large areas of bulky lymph node disease that can become painful and cause issues such as bowel obstruction. The prognosis for lymphoma is very variable and treatment options include chemotherapy, radiotherapy and surgery.

Many patients and their families have heard of Hodgkin's disease, and are aware of celebrities suffering this disease and being cured. 'Hodgkin cells' are a certain type of cell seen in one group of lymphomas and not seen in 'non-Hodgkin' lymphoma types. The 'Hodgkin' form of lymphoma is considered potentially curable. However, the classification is much more complicated than this, and 'non-Hodgkin' lymphoma includes many different types of lymphomas. These can range from slow-moving but progressive forms, which do not respond at all to chemotherapy, to rapidly progressive forms that do. Many elderly patients can live for years with a lymphoma that behaves almost like a chronic disease, while others may have a rapid and relentlessly progressive condition that does not respond to treatment and rapidly leads to death.

The symptoms of lymphoma vary greatly depending on the areas affected. The disease can, for example, arise in the brain, the skin, the eye and the gastrointestinal system. Patients therefore experience a wide variety of symptoms related to the different disease sites, as well as symptoms caused by their immune system being compromised.

Pancreatic cancer

Cancer of the pancreas is an aggressive disease. Fewer than 20% of patients diagnosed with this cancer survive the first year, and only 3% are still alive five years after diagnosis. The most common initial symptoms include abdominal pain, anorexia, weight loss and jaundice. Treatment options are combined chemotherapy and radiotherapy and also surgery, though only a small percentage of patients have diseased tissue that can be completely resected.

Pancreatic cancer has the potential to cause severe abdominal and back pain due to its location near an important bundle of nerves called the coeliac plexus. Nerve block of this area can be performed and this can be a very beneficial intervention.

Prostate cancer

Prostate cancer is a very common cancer and it has often been said that if men lived long enough they would all eventually get it. Prostate cancer is similar to breast cancer in that it can range from being a chronic, indolent disease to being a rapidly progressive and fatal disease of both younger and older men. The most common symptoms of prostate cancer are altered urinary function, including poor urine stream and dribbling. It may present with blood in the urine. It can usually, but not always, be detected by specific blood tests and a rectal examination to feel for enlargement of the gland.

Treatment for prostate cancer is effective if the cancer has not spread out of the gland, and may consist of regular monitoring only, hormone manipulation, radiotherapy and surgery. However, prostate cancer has a tendency to spread into the bone, and this involvement may become very extensive. The bone metastasis of prostate cancer can lead to complications, including pathological fractures and high blood calcium. Patients may experience severe bone pain and problems due to blood cell deficiencies (such as anaemia, bleeding and susceptibility to infection) in addition to problems with urinary function.

Skin cancer

Skin cancer is another very common malignancy, with the well-known risk factor of sun exposure, although some cancers can also arise in the very young or on non-sun-exposed skin. There are several types of skin cancers, ranging from those that can usually be managed by simple excision or cautery (such as basal cell cancers) to aggressive tumours that can metastasise to other areas such as the brain, lungs and liver. Melanoma is an aggressive form of skin cancer that is often treated with surgery, radiotherapy and specialised forms of chemotherapy.

Patients with advanced skin cancers can experience problems related to the sites of metastatic disease as well as problems associated with the skin itself, such as pain, bleeding, itching and ulceration. Advanced skin cancer can also cause psychosocial problems due to its appearance and the disfigurement caused by surgery and radiotherapy.

Cancer treatments

When a person is diagnosed with 'cancer', there is an expectation of treatment. Television shows are full of cancer patients who undergo weeks of 'chemo', lose their hair and subsequently recover. The therapeutic management of malignancy is a complex and rapidly changing part of medicine. Cancer can be treated by chemotherapy, which is managed by a medical oncologist, and by radiation therapy, which is managed by a radiation oncologist. Some patients receive one or other modality but many receive a combination of treatments. In most centres each case, including the results of complex histochemical testing on cell specimens, is presented to a clinical meeting and the best treatment option is chosen. Large multi-centre clinical trials inform the medical community about the relative risks and benefits of different treatments.

However, when dealing with advanced disease, it is important to remember that not all patients are suitable for treatment. Some treatments, particularly chemotherapy, can be onerous and may carry with them a significant burden and risk. Chemotherapy will only be offered to patients who are considered systemically strong enough, and whose level of function is adequate.

Each patient is considered carefully, regarding the type of cancer they have, where it has spread and their other medical problems. A 'cure' can only be achieved if a cancer has not metastasised (spread to other areas) and if there is a treatment available that can eradicate it. We know that many cancers metastasise in their early stages, often long before the diagnosis is made, and that patients can have 'micro-metastases' that do not show up on any current scans. This is why patients who have had cancer are often reviewed every six months, or every year, by their oncologist, even though they have been given the 'all clear'. The psychological burden of 'never really knowing it's gone' can be significant and can lead to anxiety, depression and a fixation on the signs and symptoms of possible disease.

Based on all the information gathered, patients can be offered either 'curative' treatment (aimed at disease eradication and the reduction of risk of recurrence) or 'palliative' treatment (aimed at slowing disease progression and/or improving the symptomatic burden of the disease). All healthcare professionals dealing with a patient need to be clear about the aims of the treatment they are offering. For example, it could cause great distress to discuss the palliative treatment of a man with non-small cell lung cancer that has spread to the liver in the same way that you would discuss the potentially curative treatment of a woman with a localised breast cancer.

It is very rare that a patient with metastatic disease can be cured but it is sometimes possible for very specific conditions such as testicular cancer. Patients should never be lied to regarding the potential of a particular treatment. Lying about this is not only unethical but also risks the destruction of the therapeutic relationship. Any patient undergoing treatment should have the aim of therapy, the duration of treatment, expected side-effects and the planned follow-up clearly explained and documented.

Chemotherapy

Chemotherapy consists of the administration of medications with the aim of treating cancer. Chemotherapy medications can be given either orally or intravenously. Treatment can range from the aggressive intravenous curative protocols to long-term hormonally based treatment aimed at controlling widespread metastatic disease.

It has often been said that cancer is so hard to cure because it comes from our own cells. This fact also helps to explain why many chemotherapeutic agents have so many side-effects.

Medications that poison cancer cells invariably 'poison' a percentage of normal cells as well. Chemotherapeutic agents work in varied and complex ways, including the destruction of cell deoxyribonucleic acid (DNA) and the instigation of changes aimed at causing apoptosis (programmed cell death).

Side-effects are so prevalent that they are an expected part of treatment, and protocols include medications to, for example, control nausea. Side-effects can range from unpleasant and transient to life-threatening. They vary depending on the type and dose of chemotherapy used but can include nausea and vomiting, diarrhoea, skin rashes, hair loss, kidney damage, nail changes, peripheral nerve changes (resulting in painful or numb hands and feet), weakening of the heart muscle, and damage to the bone marrow (which can lead to an inability to make vital infection-fighting cells). Many side-effects abate once treatment ceases but others, particularly the pain, numbness and tingling of peripheral nerves and damage to organs such as the heart and kidneys, can be permanent.

Some patients experience such severe treatment-related side-effects that chemotherapy is ceased. There is also a percentage of patients, albeit small, who die as a direct result of treatment. Occasionally, patients tolerate treatment unexpectedly well, and many patients can continue to take low-dose oral 'maintenance' chemotherapy for many years without side-effects.

Radiotherapy

Radiation oncologists treat malignancy with high-energy x-rays and radiation sources that destroy cancer cells. Their work is highly technical and is supported by a vital army of radiation therapists, nurses, technicians and physicists. Radiotherapy can be used as a primary, potentially curative, treatment for certain sorts of cancers (particularly lymphoma and prostate cancer), as an adjuvant treatment after surgery to reduce the risk of residual disease and metastasis, and as a palliative therapy for the management of pain and bleeding. Radiotherapy also has an important role in reducing the impingement of a malignant tumour on nerves and on the spinal cord.

Radiation protocols are determined according to the type of cancer and its location. Patients undergo extensive imaging, and an individual treatment plan is designed. Although the actual radiation delivery is brief, the majority of cancers require repeated exposure (called 'fractions') over time. For example, a man receiving aggressive treatment for prostate cancer may require treatment five days a week for six weeks, whereas a patient receiving palliative treatment for a painful metastasis to a bone may receive a single treatment.

Large machines, called linear accelerators, deliver beams to a precise location. The angling and placement of these beams is complex. Extensive efforts, often including individualised immobilisation aids such as casts and masks, are used to ensure that patients remain absolutely still during treatment. Most patients tolerate the brief duration of actual treatment well, although the hard bed around which the machine moves as it delivers the fractions can be very uncomfortable.

Patients receiving treatment for cancers in the head and neck are often required to wear a close-fitting mask during treatment and this can cause significant anxiety in susceptible individuals. Due to the nature of the treatment, the patient must be alone during the actual radiation delivery and this can exacerbate feelings of fear, anxiety and claustrophobia. The provision of low-dose relaxant medications before treatment can be beneficial. Radiation therapy carries with it a range of side-effects that vary, depending on the site being treated and the extent of the treatment. Skin redness, mouth and throat ulceration, hair loss, nausea, diarrhoea, bladder irritation and fatigue are common. Many side-effects resolve in the weeks after treatment has been completed, but scarring and fibrosis can remain.

Radiation oncologists also manage the treatment of some malignancies with a modality called 'brachytherapy', in which a radioactive seed is brought into contact with an area of internal malignancy.

Radiation therapy is a very effective treatment for the palliative management of pain caused by metastasis to bone and other tissues. It can also be used to shrink tumours and thereby assist in the palliative management of airway obstruction and venous obstruction. Bleeding from eroding skin tumours can often be successfully palliated by a single fraction of radiotherapy, and side-effects are generally non-existent. Each body tissue has a 'ceiling dose' for radiation exposure, beyond which normal tissue destruction is increasingly likely to occur. When an area has previously been treated with a curative protocol, this 'ceiling dose' limit may restrict the ability to treat the same area again in the palliative phase of care.

Chapter 7
Organ failure

Any organ can fail and many patients live for many years with heart failure and kidney failure that is managed by medications and dialysis. Eventually, however, medications can no longer support the failing organ, or it becomes clear that the burden of treatment is outweighing the benefit. The prognosis in organ failure is sometimes more difficult to predict than it is in malignancy. Patients with heart and liver failure, in particular, may follow a course of repeated exacerbations and partial recoveries. Overall, however, their condition slowly deteriorates and they can have a significant symptom burden for many years. Patients with organ failure who have exhausted curative options, or who are maximally medically managed but still symptomatic, can benefit greatly from palliative care.

Heart failure

Heart failure is the most common form of organ failure and can result from vascular disease that has caused ischaemic heart disease and infarction ('heart attacks'), from diseases or enlargement of the heart muscle itself, or from other, rarer, problems related to the heart valves and the lungs. Heart failure can also be caused by systemic illness or certain medical treatments including some forms of chemotherapy.

The symptoms of heart failure include shortness of breath, chest pain, fatigue, leg swelling and problems related to poor peripheral blood flow such as venous ulcers. Most patients with advanced heart failure are very limited in their exercise capacity. They may have to sleep propped up in bed, due to severe shortness of breath when they lie flat. These patients are at a greatly increased risk of further events such as myocardial infarction and stroke.

For many patients with end-stage heart failure, breathlessness is the most distressing symptom. Patients whose oxygen saturations are poor may find supplemental oxygen beneficial.

However, for many patients, oxygen levels are adequate but the feeling of distressing shortness of breath, or dyspnoea, remains. For these patients, the provision of a fan to move the air and the optimised management of anxiety are important. In palliative care, there is good evidence that the use of low-dose, sustained-release opiates is very beneficial for patients experiencing distressing breathlessness. This simple intervention, which is often ignored because medical practitioners only associate the use of opioids with pain relief, can provide greatly improved quality of life and a reduction in sleep deprivation, depression and anxiety.

Liver failure

The liver is a vital organ that may be damaged by malignancy, infections such as hepatitis, some medical conditions and as a result of cirrhosis due to alcohol. Most patients who have end-stage liver failure have lived with poor liver function for many years. The most common symptoms of advanced liver failure are fatigue, oedema of the lower limbs, upper abdominal pain, nausea and problems related to the fact that the liver is no longer able to produce adequate amounts of blood-clotting proteins.

In many cases, patients also experience itching, jaundice and a form of confusion known as 'hepatic encephalopathy'. This can progress to coma and death. For many patients, the symptoms of hepatic encephalopathy can be managed effectively in the community by the use of the simple laxative lactulose. This works because lactulose is very effective at helping the body expel ammonia, and it is the increased ammonia in the blood caused by liver failure that leads to encephalopathy. As people reach the end of life, worsening liver function and their inability to manage oral lactulose make this simple treatment less and less effective.

In the palliative setting, the simple provision of regular analgesia and regular anti-emetics can significantly improve a patient's quality of life. In this situation, when the stimulus for nausea and pain is constant, the provision of 'as-needed' medications is often inadequate. Ondansetron is an effective anti-emetic, which may be useful for the itch caused by the irritative effects of bile salts, whereas the antihistamines seem to have minimal effect.

Some patients with end-stage liver failure may have lived in poor socio-economic circumstances due to drug and alcohol addiction. Alcohol abuse and hepatitis C (often due to intravenous drug abuse) are common causes of this syndrome. Early referral to social workers, psychologists and drug and alcohol services can be very beneficial. However, it is important to remember that some patients with liver failure have no history of drug or alcohol use and feel stigmatised by this association. As always, it is imperative to choose your language carefully and not to make assumptions about aetiology in any patient, whatever their age, sex or social circumstances.

Kidney failure

Kidney failure has been described as an 'impending epidemic' because, as the population ages, more people are living with kidney-damaging diseases such as diabetes for longer, and healthcare systems do not have the capacity to provide dialysis for all patients living with poor renal function. There are many causes of kidney failure, including hypertension, diabetes and chronic inflammation, and large numbers of patients are maintained by dialysis. For many of these patients, there comes a time when the grinding episodes of dialysis need to become more frequent to maintain even borderline acceptability of blood chemistry. The palliative approach to care is appropriate during dialysis, as well as once dialysis ceases, although many palliative care services remain reluctant to accept patients on dialysis.

Patients with chronic kidney failure have a significant symptom burden, which often includes tiredness, fatigue, anaemia, oedema and nausea. Patients receiving dialysis also experience significant pain, and this is often under-appreciated by their primary care teams. Bone pain is common and may be severe. Many patients have had years of bi-weekly, or more frequent, dialysis and long histories of dietary and fluid intake modification, transfusions and other medications and therefore the role of 'being sick' has had a large impact on their lives. The decision to cease dialysis is one that can often be easiest for patients themselves, and much more difficult for families, carers and healthcare professionals. Patients often state that they are simply 'fed up' with dialysis and are finding that the sessions no longer provide any improvement in their quality of life.

The role of the care team in this context should be a supportive one, aimed at facilitating the patient's wishes by giving the family empathetic support. Maintaining a clear emphasis on the patient's wishes is central to this process. For example, providing evidence that red blood cell counts and creatinine are responding less and less positively to dialysis can be helpful for a family struggling to accept that a patient 'no longer wants to keep fighting'. The idea that stopping a distressing treatment is somehow 'admitting defeat' can be very damaging. Families need support to understand that the treatment that was for so long 'a lifeline' has now become an unacceptable burden.

Patients who produce a reasonable volume of urine survive much longer than those who are anuric (producing no urine), even when renal function falls to negligible levels. End-stage renal failure bestows the gift of a peaceful death in the vast majority of patients, with fatigue becoming drowsiness, then coma and finally death.

Chronic airway disease

Cigarette smoking, occupational dust and asbestos exposure, auto-immune disease, asthma and cardiovascular disease can all result in progressive respiratory failure. Patients who are maximally medically managed often approach the final stages of their life wasted, weak and bed- or wheelchair-bound. Like heart failure patients, people with advanced chronic lung diseases often follow a protracted disease course, which is marked by exacerbations and partial recoveries.

Oxygen has been found to be a valuable intervention for people who are hypoxic (having low oxygen saturations, usually taken as below 90%) on room air. However, most people with end-stage respiratory failure end up on domiciliary oxygen, despite the fact that medical air seems to be equally effective if hypoxia is not present. In end-stage respiratory disease, morphine has been shown to be the most beneficial intervention to counteract the feeling of breathlessness that the majority of patients describe as the most distressing part of their illness. However, many clinicians are only familiar with prescribing opioid medications for pain. It is therefore imperative to find a prescriber who is familiar with managing breathlessness in the palliative setting.

A feeling of breathlessness can result in a pervasive feeling of panic and a fear of suffocation. Anxiety becomes a major issue for many patients, leading to a vicious cycle of anxiety and breathlessness that may require sedative medication. Many patients benefit from simple interventions – like improved air flow, a fan or open window, energy-sparing techniques for mobility that can often by optimised by an occupational therapist or physiotherapist, and medication to control depression and anxiety.

Some patients have been managed with an extensive regime of inhaled agents for many years. As they lose their ability to inhale properly, these medications become less effective, and inhaled salbutamol ('ventolin', used for asthma) may worsen anxiety as it can cause increased heart rates.

Patients whose breathlessness and anxiety cannot be managed using the measures described above should be commenced on titrated doses of opioids. If symptom control is still poor and the patient is distressed, sedation may be needed. At this stage, management in a tertiary palliative care unit or an acute hospital is generally warranted.

Chapter 8
Neurodegenerative disorders

The neurodegenerative disorders most often seen in generalist palliative care settings are motor neurone disease, multiple sclerosis and Parkinson's disease. However, a patient may also experience progressive neurological dysfunction for many other reasons, particularly as a result of stroke and substance use.

Motor neurone disease (MND)

MND is also referred to as amyotrophic lateral sclerosis (ALS), Lou Gehrig's Disease, SLA (from the French translation of ALS – sclerose laterale amyotrophique) and Charcot's disease. There are many forms of MND, often differentiated by whether they affect the section of the nerve that travels from the spinal cord down to the end tissue or the area of nerve that travels from the cord up to the brain. Some forms affect the areas of the mouth, face and throat severely, whereas other forms initially affect other areas such as the legs and arms. The great majority of cases of MND occur without a known cause.

The symptoms of MND result from its effect on the innervation of muscle. They may include weakness, muscle twitching, loss of muscle mass, rigidness and stiffness of muscles, speech problems and depression. Many patients experience trouble swallowing and require a PEG tube for artificial feeding.

There is no treatment for MND and the symptoms are relentlessly progressive. Many patients die within a couple of years of diagnosis at best. In the final stages of the disease, the patient is often unable to move voluntarily at all and progressive loss of the muscles of respiration eventually results in death. MND is a devastating disease that can affect previously healthy people in their twenties, thirties and forties as well as older people. The principal challenges include managing these patients' often severe psycho-spiritual distress and providing the intense nursing care required for positioning.

Patients with MND require a multidisciplinary approach from nursing, medical, occupational therapy, psychology and physiotherapy professionals. Due to their inability to move when they are uncomfortable, these patients are at high risk of developing pressure sores. Customised positioning inserts and splinting are vital. Medications can be utilised to ease pain and manage muscle spasms and nausea. They may need referral to specialist medical practitioners, such as neurologists, to provide injections to assist in drying up embarrassing and distressing saliva. In the final stages of life, many patients require continuous analgesic and anxiolytic medications.

It is very important to remember that many patients with MND retain their intellectual function until very late in their disease course. Most patients lose the ability to speak quite early on, and the provision of individualised communication aids is beneficial for both the patients and the carers.

Multiple sclerosis (MS)

MS is an inflammatory disease that leads to damage of the protective layer around the nerves. The damage results in nerves becoming unable to communicate with each other properly. MS is a very variable disease that can progress relentlessly or in discrete episodes. It may be chronic and mild or rapidly progressive and severe.

The symptoms of MS are similarly variable. Patients may experience issues such as visual disturbance or loss of vision, weakness, clumsiness, tremor, numbness of an area and cognitive problems. The variability of symptoms, and the fact that they may 'come and go', often leads to a delay in diagnosis. In many cases, the effects of attacks may initially resolve completely but, as the disease progresses, permanent neurological problems occur.

Most patients eventually develop persisting cognitive and physical disability. There is no cure for MS but medications can be used to ease the severity of disease flares. Many patients may experience an additional symptom burden related to the prolonged use of steroid medications utilised to modify their disease. These symptoms can include thin skin, bruising, loss of muscle strength in the upper arms and legs, fluid accumulation, central obesity and susceptibility to infection.

Parkinson's disease

Parkinson's disease is a degenerative disease of the central nervous system. Cells in an area of the midbrain (called the substantia nigra) die, and abnormal deposits of protein accumulate.

Most cases of Parkinson's disease occur without a known cause. The early symptoms of the disease include alterations in gait, such as shuffling or unsteadiness, shaking, rigidity, slowing of movements and trouble writing, sleep disturbance and emotional lability. Later in the disease, behavioural problems become more common and dementia is a feature of the final stages.

Medications are effective in managing the early stages, particularly the movement-related problems of tremor and gait disturbance. Eventually, however, medications become less effective and problems related to their use (such as involuntary restlessness and uncontrolled movements) occur.

Parkinson's disease can affect adults of any age, but it is much more common in the elderly. Many diseases can produce a 'Parkinsonian syndrome' that is often indistinguishable from Parkinson's disease itself. The results of repeated minor brain trauma, as seen in boxers, are a well-known example of this.

The behavioural and emotional effects of Parkinson's disease are variable but can be a significant cause of distress for patients themselves and especially for their families and carers. Many families talk about the 'multiple losses' of neurodegenerative diseases like Parkinson's disease. They feel grief at diagnosis, and the inevitable grief when the person dies, but they also experience a prolonged grief over the loss of 'the real person'. Over time, families find it harder to recognise the person they love, as the effects of behavioural disturbance, cognitive decline, medications, processes of dementia and personality changes worsen. The services of a psychologist and disease-specific counsellors, if available, can be very beneficial.

Chapter 9

The rise of chronic disease and the 'oldest old'

We often read about the 'tsunami' of aging that is set to engulf the world's richest countries. While many developing countries struggle to feed their people and childhood death from malnutrition is common, people in developed countries are struggling with a healthcare burden largely caused by the successes of modern medicine and by our own excessive consumption. Type 2 diabetes, high blood pressure, high blood cholesterol, cigarette smoking and obesity bestow a legacy of chronic disease. Meanwhile, modern medicine ensures that people often live for many, many years with significant symptoms that, in the recent past, would have caused their death at a much younger age.

The burden of chronic disease

Most healthcare workers spend much of their time dealing with elderly patients who are living with joint pain, obesity, chronic respiratory compromise and the stigmata of atherosclerotic (narrowed blood vessels) vascular disease. Similarly, few healthcare workers are unaware of the difficulty of achieving even tiny gains in the struggle to convince patients that stopping smoking, modifying food and alcohol intake and beginning to exercise will benefit them more than simply taking yet another medication.

Many diseases that used to cause death have now become chronic diseases instead. Chronic obstructive pulmonary disease (for example, emphysema), chronic kidney disease, heart failure, some forms of myeloma, indolent forms of prostate and breast cancer and diabetes can now often be managed in the community. When these patients finally move into assisted living or old people's homes, their disease burden is therefore very high.

Accepting that medicine has its limits

Optimal supportive care can do much to ensure that people with chronic disease have the best quality of life possible but it is also important to remember that people should always be encouraged to take active responsibility for their own health. For many patients, and their families, who have lived with chronic disease for many years, the realisation that medicine has little further to offer is difficult to accept. In a society where inhalers can ameliorate the breathlessness caused by smoking, oral hypoglycaemic medications and insulin can manage the diabetes often caused by dietary excess, and anti-inflammatory medications can ease the painful knees resulting from obesity, many patients are amazed when they are told that their worsening symptoms are beyond medical control. Patients for whom the palliative approach is appropriate can feel 'abandoned' by medical practitioners and these patients may seek to apportion blame elsewhere for their situation.

When dealing with a patient's feeling of abandonment, it is important to provide both empathy and compassion. But it is equally important to refrain from criticising other members of the healthcare profession or colluding with patients in their desire to apportion blame. If a breach of the duty of care has occurred, it is of course appropriate to advocate for a patient. However, agreeing with a patient's inappropriate feelings of abandonment simply because it is 'easier' only reinforces their status as 'a helpless victim of their illness'. The advice of a clinical psychologist, psychiatrist, counsellor or pastoral care worker can be invaluable in maintaining a vital therapeutic alliance in this often difficult situation.

Social attitudes to aging

Although age itself must never be considered a disease, our society is persistently ageist. Western society is obsessed with 'staying young' and this is illustrated by the ever-increasing sales of hair dye and anti-wrinkle cream. Not surprisingly, older sections of society can feel a profound sense of disenfranchisement. Western attitudes often stand in stark contrast to the respect afforded to the elderly in many Eastern cultures, for example. In Western society, many elderly people feel as though they are 'on the scrap heap' and this is a particular issue for patients who may be socially isolated, have outlived their spouse or a child, or who have always defined their worth in society by their achievements. A man who worked hard all his life and was proud of his carpentry skills, but is distant from his children and grandchildren, may face aging with more difficulty than a woman who has devoted her life to raising children and sees a legacy in her grandchildren. Alternatively, the same woman may have taken great pride in her appearance and perhaps finds it impossible to bear the changes that inevitably come with aging. Aging can bring a huge range of responses, from contented and grateful acceptance to resentment, frustration and fear.

In services that have the necessary financial resources, the provision of therapist intervention to enable continuing participation in the activities of daily life, suitable leisure activities and to facilitate excursions out of the main care premises can be enormously helpful. Activities centred on legacy-building can be particularly beneficial. For example, assistance to write memoirs, prepare a book of favourite recipes or complete a craft project to pass down to a grandchild may enable patients to redefine their view of the aging process.

The 'oldest old'

The 'oldest old' are more usefully defined by their functional status, rather than by their chronology. After all, some people are functionally 'old' at 65 and others remain remarkably 'young' at 90. People at the extreme of functional age are sometimes bed-bound and take only small amounts of oral nourishment. They are perhaps non-verbal or at least hypophonic (having minimal speech) and have cachexia, weakness and perhaps limb contractures. Some members of this group may have end-stage dementia but it is important to consider that cognition may also be relatively well preserved in some of the 'oldest old'.

For many of these patients, it will be very beneficial to assume that they suffer 'bed ache' and provide simple analgesia such as liquid paracetamol or a transdermal patch. Staff must be encouraged to consider non-verbal cues indicating pain and to take note of, and importantly record, signs such as restlessness, agitation, facial grimaces, altered vocalisation and altered posturing. In many cases, a trial of gentle analgesia and careful documentation will be of immense benefit.

Medical practitioners are sometimes reluctant to order pain relief for patients who do not appear to be in pain. However, any patient confined to bed will confirm that they become very uncomfortable, and any patient unable to change their own position at will is particularly susceptible to joint and muscle pain, contractures and pressure effects. The optimal management of bed-bound patients includes pressure care, regular turning, bladder and bowel management, mouth care and gentle analgesia titrated to effect.

Chapter 10

Recognising and treating the dying patient

Many poor care outcomes in general medical wards result from the failure to diagnose dying. Medical practitioners are adept at diagnosing a huge variety of illnesses, but clear signs that the end of life is close are often missed, misinterpreted or ignored. Failure to diagnose dying leads to burdensome, expensive and futile testing and medication and to a lack of comfort- and dignity-focused care. In addition, families and carers are not afforded the privilege of knowing that death is close.

What are the signs that death is getting closer?

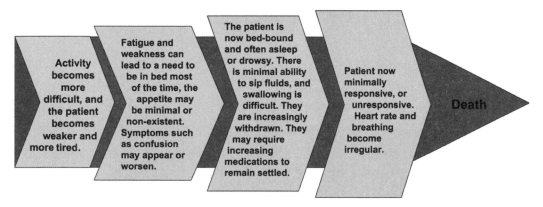

Figure 10.1 *What are the signs that death is getting closer?*

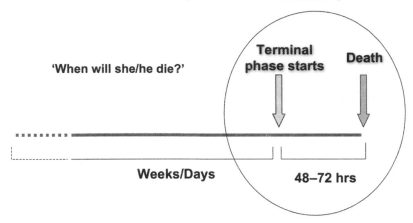

Figure 10.2 *Identifying the terminal phase*

The ability to diagnose the dying phase not only allows healthcare staff to provide optimal care, but also allows those closest to the patient to adjust to their impending death. It provides time to say any last things that have perhaps been left unsaid, to inform relatives who may wish to visit, and to make any culturally specific arrangements that may be required. Healthcare staff also benefit from the 'diagnosis of dying', as it enables them to relax their adherence to the usual aims of 'diagnosis, treatment and cure' and instead embrace the holistic, palliative care of the patient.

Diagnosing dying

Diagnosing dying is not an exact science. Whilst it is often possible to estimate how long a person will live, it should only ever be an estimate – not a forecast. The more precise a prediction, the more wrong it could end up being. It is also possible to get the diagnosis of dying wrong (and find the patient suddenly recovering), but there are some signs that are reasonably reliable.

The first aspect to consider is the patient's disease and their disease phase. Secondly, you need to look at their disease trajectory, and finally the presence (or otherwise) of the specific symptoms of the dying phase. Any patient with an advanced disease who was previously functioning adequately, who has had a period of deterioration unresponsive to medical measures, and for whom the situation is irreversible and now presents with some, or all, of the following is likely (but not definitely!) to be in the dying phase:

- Drowsiness or coma
- The inability to get out of bed
- Verbal interaction restricted to a few words or less
- The ability to take only sips of fluid
- A persisting delirium
- New and persisting or worsening dyspnoea (breathlessness)

In previously debilitated patients, the situation may be less clear, but any debilitated patient with a new and progressive infection or the development of persisting shortness of breath, delirium or a reduced level of consciousness is also likely to be dying

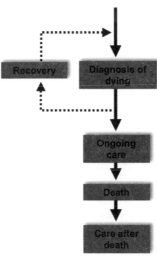

It is possible to get the diagnosis of dying wrong!

Figure 10.3 *Palliative care may not always follow the expected course*

Managing the 'dying phase'

The 'dying phase' is generally considered to last anything from a few hours to a few days. The diagnosis of the dying phase should not only prompt discussions with family members but should also lead seamlessly to a review of care provision. This review consists of five simple steps:

- Medication review and cessation of all non-essential medications

- Provision of terminal care medications for the management of pain, nausea, secretions and agitation, using an appropriate route of administration
- Provision of routine mouth and eye care
- Ensuring the management of urination, either by indwelling catheter or by bladder scanning, to ensure that retention does not occur
- The cessation of further invasive testing

Patients who are dying are unable to swallow reliably, so it is best for medications to be provided by continuous 'as needed' subcutaneous infusion. Urinary obstruction is most common in men but can occur in any patient. It is easily diagnosed by palpation and can be confirmed by bladder scan. A distended bladder can cause agitation, and can be simply managed by insertion of an indwelling catheter. The simple provision of saliva substitute and lubricating eye drops can also greatly increase comfort in the terminal phase.

Talking to family members about death

Many staff, especially those who only rarely deal with patients in the terminal phase, find it hard to start a conversation with family members or carers. However, it is important to remember that many families are well aware of the situation and may be waiting for healthcare staff to initiate a discussion. Asking open questions to elicit the opinions of families and carers, whilst also providing some hint as to your own perspective, can be a valuable first step:

> 'Things have changed a great deal in the last few days, haven't they? How do you think your mum is today?'

> 'I was surprised at how much more unwell Joan was today when I saw her, compared to yesterday… Do you think things are changing more quickly now?'

> 'It is my feeling that Fred is deteriorating very quickly now. What do you think?'

> 'Unfortunately it seems as though the antibiotics have had no effect. Shirley seems much less responsive today. What do you think?'

In many cases, families and carers will come to their own conclusion that death is close but sometimes it is important to say things clearly (see Chapter 5):

> 'We often look at how fast things are changing. If you notice changes in your dad's condition every month, then things are changing slowly, but in this case things are changing every day. I think he is a lot weaker and drowsier than he was yesterday and I think time is growing very short. Do you feel that he is reaching the end of his life?'

'We often see changes like those Sally is experiencing, as death gets closer. I think she may be getting close to the time when she is going to die.'

'I have just been with Dr Brown and we saw John. Dr Brown has decided to change some of the medications and to make sure that there are extra doses of medications available for end of life care because it seems that he will die quite soon.'

Many care providers express concern about using the words 'die' and 'death' in conversations with family. Whilst each situation is different, it is generally true that a gentle but clear conversation that is not open to misinterpretation is of most benefit. Extreme emotions are always liable to alter people's ability to process difficult concepts and convoluted language. Needing to rely on interpretation, suggestion or innuendo is very unwise. Yet many healthcare workers are surprised when a statement that they had thought was clear is misconstrued by a distressed family.

Weakness and fatigue

Weakness and fatigue, as well as cachexia (see p. 68), are very important symptoms in recognising the dying patient and require careful treatment by care providers. Weakness and tiredness are some of the most pervasive symptoms of serious illness. Patients with cancer or advanced organ failure describe an almost overwhelming sense of fatigue, and it is certainly a debilitating symptom that erodes both quality of life and sense of personal worth. It is often beneficial to explain, in simple terms, that metastatic malignancy and organ failure cause weakness and fatigue. Many patients blame themselves, and are indeed blamed, by family members, who may go so far as to say that the patient is 'lazy' or 'not trying'. Careful discussion of the impact of malignancy and the altered physiology resulting from metabolic imbalance, as well as the burden of treatment, can be very helpful.

Medications are sometimes prescribed in order to improve fatigue, notably the steroid dexamethasone and some stimulant drugs. However, these have significant potential side-effects. Prescriptions need to be individualised and patients carefully monitored. The results are very variable and, even if beneficial, temporary. The most beneficial interventions tend to involve counselling as part of a palliative approach to care.

Patients who have always defined themselves by their employment, physical skill or strength have a particularly difficult time managing fatigue. They rapidly come to believe that they are 'useless' and a 'burden' and may experience profound depression as a result of poor self-worth. Care providers can assist by gently, and often repeatedly, reinforcing two simple concepts: the first is that the illness is to blame, not the person; and the second is that we are more than we do. Referral to social work, pastoral care or psychology professionals may also be very helpful.

> 'I know you're feeling really fed up, Brian. People often tell me that the weakness and tiredness is impossible to describe. I want you to make sure that you always remember that it's the cancer that is to blame. That's the reason you feel so dreadful – can you try and remember that and not blame yourself?'

> 'I know you're struggling with the fact that you can't get out and do all the things you used to be able to do. It must be really frustrating but just try and remember that you are much more to your family than simply a farmer. There's still a lot you can give and, although you may not be able to jump on the tractor, you can still talk to your grandchildren and pass on a whole lot of valuable information.'

Some patients may benefit greatly from an opportunity to engage in appropriate legacy-building and in Australia and New Zealand this can often be facilitated by a diversional therapist. These therapists can assist the patient with writing out some recipes, recording some life stories or painting a simple card. This may enable a person who is too fatigued to undertake normal activity the opportunity to complete an affirming task.

However, for some patients, the burden of weakness and fatigue can be almost overwhelming. It is difficult to generalise about the type of patients most affected but high-achieving, career-driven men, and men who have always prided themselves on being physically active, strong and virile, are at increased risk. Men from cultures that emphasise the concepts of masculinity and physical strength may also struggle, often silently, with their new situation. For a parent or spouse who has always taken pride in their ability to provide, having to be the receiver of care (rather than the giver of care) can be intolerable. For patients like these, no amount of counselling may be able to refocus their self-worth onto concepts of interpersonal interaction. Assessment by a psychologist and, if necessary, referral to a psychiatrist may be needed.

Cachexia

Advanced cancer is often signalled by muscle wasting and weight loss. It is valuable to carefully explain to patients and their families that cancer itself causes progressive weight loss and a lack of appetite. Many family members blame themselves for the fact that a patient does not wish to eat, and patients themselves may experience guilt over their lack of interest in food.

In the palliative setting, it is right to encourage people to simply eat 'what they feel like, when they feel like it'. A dietician review and the provision of supplements may be perfectly appropriate and beneficial in situations such as continuing chemotherapy or progression to rehabilitation. However, in the palliative phase the body is unable to make any use of dense nutrition. Any benefit will be more than outweighed by the potential for nausea, and the loss of opportunity to enjoy a favourite food instead.

Families may benefit from advice on how to involve the patient in the socially important routines of mealtimes in ways that remove any emphasis on the amount eaten. Small servings, frequent small snacks rather than large meals, and the provision of moist and cool foods, such as custards and ice creams, can be helpful. (See the section in Chapter 11 on 'Appetite loss, hydration and nutrition', page 71.)

Cachexia carries with it not only a glaringly evident reminder of serious illness, but also its own symptom burden. The loss of 'padding' leads to worsening joint pain and predisposes patients to developing pressure sores. Weakness and frailty progress – in line with worsening cachexia – and patients often develop extra discomforts caused by severe and rapid weight loss, such as ill-fitting dentures and the annoying 'noises in the ear' caused by Eustachian tube dysfunction.

Chapter 11

Medical treatment versus medical care

The concepts of care versus treatment vary across the globe. In many countries, medical staff are required to provide care but are not always legally required to treat. It is important for all healthcare staff to familiarise themselves with the situation in their own healthcare system. Providing a dying patient with pain relief, warmth and personal hygiene is regarded as 'care', whereas providing intravenous antibiotics or surgery, for example, is 'treatment'. In many countries, medical staff have the right to decline to offer treatment when they feel that such treatment would be unlikely to be effective and/or would cause unacceptable burden or risk of harm.

When difficult decisions have to be made and conflict may arise, it can be very valuable to consult clinicians experienced in health law and ethics. Most large hospitals have these experts and they can often give insightful advice over the telephone.

Appetite loss, hydration and nutrition

As described previously, loss of appetite is very common in the advanced stages of serious illness, especially malignancy. In this situation, it is common for families to ask questions regarding the provision of artificial hydration and nutrition. This is an area that can cause great distress for many carers and healthcare professionals and is also an area where treatment paradigms vary depending on cultural and religious beliefs. There is no simple answer to the question of how best to manage end-stage dehydration and malnutrition, but there are several points to bear in mind as guidelines when developing individualised approaches.

Firstly, it is important to be clear that, in this instance, the issues for a patient suffering advanced malignancy are not the same as for a patient with, for example, multiple sclerosis. Patients with metastatic malignancy, who have reached the palliative phase of care, can no longer utilise or metabolise nutrients normally. It is therefore pointless to give them supplemental nutrition. In fact, the nutrients may boost the growth rate of the cancer, and at worst they will create nausea, diarrhoea, abdominal pain, an increased risk of aspiration and added care cost. The focus for family can easily become the nutrition, rather than the patient themselves. For these patients 'what you feel like, when you feel like it' remains the best approach.

For other patients, without the issue of malignancy, the situation is more complex. In these cases, it is important to consider the patient's wishes, the aim of nutrition, and how likely it is to be achieved, and quality of life. A patient with motor neurone disease may choose to continue PEG feeding in order to optimise the chances of prolonged survival at home but may, just as legitimately, decide to cease supplemental feeding when they are in hospital and approaching the final stages of their life. Similarly, a patient with advanced heart failure may choose to abide carefully by a supplemented diet with the aim of improving nutritional status but may also decide to take only desired amounts of chosen foods in order to maximise enjoyment.

In some centres, it is considered best practice to provide small amounts of supplemental fluid, usually via the subcutaneous route, right through the terminal phase. In other units, patients are offered desired oral intake only. Families often express the fear that patients will 'die of dehydration' and it is important that care teams are confident about discussing this issue. Dying patients are, as nature intended, dehydrated. Patients very, very rarely complain of thirst, although they frequently complain of a dry mouth. Many families and carers confuse the two. Providing saliva substitute, and encouraging frequent swabbing of the mouth with cool water and regular application of lip balm, will usually provide comfort.

Overly enthusiastic supplemental fluids can result in nausea, vomiting, subcutaneous site pooling, oedema, ascites, pulmonary oedema and increased cardiovascular stress. Careful and gentle provision of fluid may, however, provide a heightened feeling of well-being. It is important to repeatedly, if necessary, remind the family of the reason for the patient's inability to drink naturally. It is easy for them to start focusing simply on hydration, and by extension on the volume of that hydration, and for the role of an advanced cancer to be ignored.

'Tom, I know you are concerned that Arthur is not drinking enough but it is important to remember that his body can no longer manage fluids properly. If we poured large

amounts of fluid into a vein, I'm afraid it would all leak out into the tissues of his arms and legs or pool in his lungs or abdomen. It wouldn't do what you are hoping it would do because the cancer has made it impossible for his liver and kidneys to manage. We will make sure his mouth and lips are kept moist, and of course he can have a drink if he wants one at any time. '

'Lisa, it's important to remember that all of Elsie's organs are now affected by her liver failure. Everything is beginning to shut down and I'm afraid that increasing the fluids through the vein will only create more of a strain on her heart and kidneys. I know it's difficult because you and I are always told to drink more water but the situation is very different when someone is so sick.'

'I know that you are hoping that increasing the fluids will help Bob but I'm afraid the cancer is too advanced. We need to remember that all of his organs are starting to shut down now and his body simply cannot process the added fluid like you or I could. He can have whatever he likes by mouth and we are happy to continue the small amount that we are giving under the skin but his body simply can't manage more than that. I think that pushing lots of extra fluids through a vein might do more harm than good, and it could leak into his lungs or abdomen and make things worse.'

'I know that both you and Toby are very worried that Toby can no longer drink enough. Toby, we are happy to try some gentle and slow subcutaneous fluids for a few days, to see if that makes you feel better. But if it doesn't help, I think we should stop and concentrate on other ways to make sure you are comfortable.'

It is important to remember that the offering or provision of food and drink is fundamental to the way that we show care. In some cases, family members will be unable to accept advice that a dying family member does not require hydration. In this instance, it is far preferable to offer the option of gentle subcutaneous fluid therapy, rather than risk a breakdown of the therapeutic alliance at such a critical time. Intravenous cannulation can be traumatic and is painful and unnecessary in the terminal phase. In contrast, subcutaneous fluids run at a rate of 40–60ml per hour, will rarely cause local skin or tissue problems, and will often provide a great deal of solace to a grieving family.

Symptom control

When we consider symptom control in the palliative phase of care, there are three important points to keep in mind. The first is that, when treatment and cure are impossible, symptom control assumes greater significance. The second is that the experience of many symptoms, especially pain, is influenced by several other factors such as psycho-spiritual distress and family disharmony. The third is that it is vitally important to be honest about what medications can achieve. It is inappropriate and unhelpful to promise total freedom from pain to a man with widespread bone metastasis and spinal fracture, when the best that can actually be hoped for is comfort at rest and tolerable discomfort when mobilising. Scrupulous attention to symptom complexes on history, and careful review of the effect of any intervention, are cornerstones of the palliative approach.

Nausea and vomiting

Nausea and vomiting are two different symptoms that may have different causes. They are very common, especially in patients with a malignancy, and can cause a level of distress commensurate with pain. Several studies have shown that these symptoms are greatly feared and poorly managed in many patients.

Nausea and vomiting have numerous possible causes. Structural abnormality or irritation of any part of the gastrointestinal tract can cause abdominal pain, nausea and vomiting. Abnormal function of the stomach and gut can result in slowing of peristalsis (normal propulsive movements) and lead to gastric stasis, and any significant abnormality in the chemical environment of the body can also result in these symptoms. Raised intracranial pressure and medication- or treatment-related side-effects are also common causes of nausea and vomiting.

In any patient, it is important to try to determine the cause of nausea and vomiting, although this can often be difficult. A careful history may reveal an association with, for example, radiotherapy, chemotherapy or a new medication. The relationship of the symptoms to oral intake and bowel movements may indicate gastric stasis, reflux, constipation or abdominal colic caused by an abdominal mass. Examination may suggest the presence of a cerebral lesion, an enlarged liver leading to compression of the stomach, ascitic fluid, an abdominal mass or symptoms consistent with a bowel obstruction.

Review of blood tests may reveal liver or renal impairment, deranged electrolytes or increased calcium. In a few patients, the cause of nausea and vomiting is reversible. Hypercalcaemia is an example of a rapidly reversible cause of nausea. Often, simply introducing an anti-acid medication is very beneficial. However, in many patients in the palliative phase, it is the underlying disease that causes nausea and vomiting. In this situation, judicious and appropriate medication is required.

There are multiple anti-emetics available. The choice of drug is usually based on the proposed mechanism of the nausea, although the use of broad-spectrum anti-emetics is increasing. Bowel obstruction caused by malignant disease is relatively common in the terminal phase, particularly in ovarian and bowel cancer. On rare occasions, a patient may be suitable for surgical intervention and this should be rapidly facilitated if appropriate.

Often, however, bowel obstruction heralds the beginning of the terminal phase. Research continues into the optimal treatment of obstruction in the palliative phase, but the use of some combination of dexamethasone, ranitidine, ondansetron and octreotide is usually indicated. Nasogastric (NG) tubes are the mainstay of decompressive treatment of obstruction in the acute setting and can be very useful for rapidly controlling vomiting. Their prolonged use in palliative care is controversial, as they can be distressing and undignified. Some patients may tolerate them well but the majority of patients are best managed without a NG tube and with a continuous subcutaneous infusion.

When nausea and vomiting are caused by raised intracranial pressure, the steroid dexamethasone is the main treatment. However, when nausea and vomiting have other causes, the medication choice is less well defined. Whichever medication is chosen, it is important that it is given regularly and by the appropriate route and that the effectiveness of the treatment and development of any side-effects are assessed. Many patients whose nausea and vomiting is poorly managed are found to be receiving only 'as needed' anti-emetics by the oral route. They usually settle quickly when regular anti-emetics via the subcutaneous route are commenced, their medication regime is reviewed, and drugs known to cause nausea (such as some lipid lowering drugs and oral anti-inflammatory medications) are ceased.

Commonsense advice regarding the choice of small, simple meals, the avoidance of caffeine, alcohol, highly spiced foods and cigarette smoking, and the appropriate management of constipation, is vital. Uncontrolled nausea and vomiting is a reason for admission to hospital and, if required, admission to a tertiary palliative care unit.

Anxiety and depression

The symptom of anxiety covers a wide spectrum, from common anxiety associated with stress to the disabling anxiety of a panic attack.

'Simple' anxiety is part of many people's lives, and second only to depression as a cause of psychiatric morbidity. The palliative phase is not the time to attempt to 'cure' a long-standing anxiety disorder! Symptoms such as breathlessness and pain may worsen pre-existing anxiety or result in new anxiety. In either case, it is important to be aware of the pre-morbid function of the patient and of any significant history, such as previous depression or suicidal impulses. Professional support from a psychiatrist or psychologist can be very helpful. Techniques such as relaxation, meditation and cognitive behavioural therapy can be highly effective in some people and completely ineffective in others.

Optimised management of other symptoms, appropriate social and spiritual support and the commencement of a low-dose anti-depressant are often beneficial initial interventions. For many patients in the palliative phase, sedative medications such as the benzodiazepines may be required. Patients and families may require careful counselling as to the benefits of these drugs regarding the management of disabling or distressing anxiety versus their fears of addiction. Dependence is not as great an issue for patients in a palliative care phase as it is, for example, for patients in rehabilitation, and monitored benzodiazepine use is preferable to self-medication with alcohol and other drugs.

Careful introduction, titration and monitoring are important. It is also vital that the patient, family and care provider are all educated regarding the development of dependence and the need for very gradual withdrawal if the medication is ceased.

Panic attacks are a severe form of episodic anxiety that can occur suddenly. They can be extremely frightening and disabling, and review by a mental health professional is important. 'As needed' benzodiazepines are usually the treatment of choice.

Depression is common in patients during the palliative phase of care, just as it is at other times in life. However, care must be taken to differentiate normal feelings of sadness, loss and grief from true depression. Patients and their families need to be encouraged to discuss their feelings about severe illness and approaching death. However, rapid labelling of a patient as 'depressed' simply because they are sad is inappropriate and unhelpful. Often, asking the simple question 'Do you feel you are depressed?' is the best way of ascertaining the presence of depression, as distinct from appropriate sadness.

True depression can often be recognised by pervasive feelings of sadness that remove the ability to enjoy previously enjoyable activities, disturbance of sleep and appetite and a feeling of worthlessness. Some studies have shown that a feeling of worthlessness (as distinct from sadness, tiredness or loneliness) is a good indicator of clinical depression in this patient group. Review by a mental health professional is beneficial and the introduction of low-dose anti-depressant medication often leads to improvement. Any patient whose depression worsens with first-line treatment must be reviewed by a psychiatrist, as there are several mental health disorders (particularly bipolar disorder) that can be exacerbated by anti-depressants. These disorders require specialist anti-psychotic medications that primary healthcare providers may be unfamiliar with.

Delirium and agitation

Delirium is an altered state of mental alertness and functioning that is characterised by sudden or recent onset, and fluctuating character. There are many causes of delirium, including infection, electrolyte imbalance and constipation. It is useful to consider the concept of 'vulnerability versus insult'. An invulnerable patient may develop delirium if the insult is significant enough – for example, a young man developing confusion due to post-operative infection. A highly vulnerable individual may develop delirium with minimal insult – for example, an elderly man with cancer who becomes constipated. A delirious patient is intermittently or variably confused and disorientated, with altered behaviour, and may experience hallucinations. The diagnosis can be difficult, especially in patients with dementia, and an awareness of baseline function is therefore important.

Delirium is common in the palliative phase, and increasingly common as death approaches. In this patient group, the cause is often multifactorial, and fewer patients have a reversible cause for their delirium when compared to general hospital patients. Delirium falls into three categories: hypoactive, hyperactive and mixed. Patients with hyperactive delirium are typically reviewed early because they are calling out, trying to get out of bed, repeatedly reaching out and plucking or removing blankets. They may also be verbally (and occasionally physically) aggressive. Patients with hypoactive delirium are more easily missed, as they may simply sit quietly and appear vague and disorientated. This form of delirium is often confused with depression.

Patients with cancer can develop a form of meningitis, due to seeding of the covering of the brain and spinal cord with cancer cells. This 'neoplastic meningitis' can present with a wide variety of neurological changes, but can also present with delirium, confusion and behavioural changes.

A delirious patient should be thoroughly assessed for reversible factors. However, in the terminal phase this is often inappropriate. It is important for the care team to consider the situation for the individual patient and analyse the potential findings of each proposed test and consider whether a result will change management. Palliative patients who have recovered from a period of delirium often, but not always, recall it as frightening and confusing. For this reason, it is always important to assess even the frailest patient. Treatment of infection, management of urinary retention, medication review and the cessation of potentially problematic medications (especially those with an anti-cholinergic load) is appropriate. All patients should have their delirium managed. Haloperidol, olanzapine and risperidone are the most frequently used medications.

Agitation is frequently seen in the terminal phase. Usually, it can be easily managed using optimal pain control and low-dose and carefully titrated benzodiazepines either subcutaneously (for example, midazolam or clonazepam) or sublingually (for example, clonazepam). It is important to check that there is no occult cause, such as urinary retention, for any new agitation.

Terminal agitation (a subset of delirium) is a severe form of agitation that appears in the final hours or days of life. Terminal agitation often requires the use of high-dose benzodiazepine, and in extreme cases may require the introduction of drugs such as phenobarbitone or levomepromazine. It is a reason for inpatient care and may require terminal sedation and admission to a tertiary palliative care unit.

Blood sugar management

The enthusiasm with which blood sugar levels should be regulated must be considered in the context of the whole patient. The issues for a newly diagnosed diabetic aged 30 with no end-organ damage are very different from those in an 80-year-old man with diabetic-related kidney disease, visual loss and peripheral neuropathy. It is far preferable for palliative patients to have sugars that are slightly high, rather than risk the collapse and falls that can come with low blood sugar. Very high sugars (for example, over 20) can lead to increased infections, polyuria, headache and nausea. The burden of multiple oral agents, frequent insulin injections and repeated testing may be excessive. It is therefore often appropriate to have a once-daily slow-release insulin and daily random testing, with the aim of maintaining sugars above 5 and below 15.

Dyspnoea

Dyspnoea is breathlessness. The sensation of air hunger (and the increased work and effort of breathing) is a disabling symptom that is often associated with the advanced stages of heart failure, chronic airways disease and lung cancer. Patients with any disorder that affects the muscles of respiration (such as motor neurone disease and malignant cachexia) can also experience breathlessness. Recurrent pleural effusion is a common cause of breathlessness in palliative care. Draining of an effusion can provide rapid relief but repeated drainage should be carefully reviewed with regard to the rapidity of re-accumulation and the degree of benefit.

It is fundamentally frightening to feel at risk of suffocation, and many patients experience severe associated anxiety and panic.

Research indicates that oxygen is only beneficial if the patient is hypoxic (saturation levels below 90%) on room air but increased air flow, whether from a fan or nasal air, can be beneficial for all patients (Abernethy, McDonald, *et al.* 2010).

Optimal management of pain and anxiety is important and many patients can benefit from learning relaxation and breathing exercises. Techniques for energy conservation and optimised provision of aids can be managed by a combination of occupational therapy and physiotherapy.

Slow-release morphine has been studied and found to be of significant benefit for the management of dyspnoea (Abernethy, Currow, *et al.* 2003) and should be instituted for disabling breathlessness even when the patient is free of pain. The maxim 'start low and go slow' is applicable in this situation and when prescribing for pain. It is also worth remembering that whoever prescribes opioids should also prescribe the required laxatives. Severe and unmanageable dyspnoea is an indication for admission to an inpatient unit and may necessitate tertiary palliative care management.

Dry mouth

As mentioned in the previous section on 'Appetite loss, hydration and nutrition' (pages 71– 73), complaints of dry mouth are far more frequent than those of thirst. Many of the drugs frequently used in the palliative phase of care – for example, the opioids, and common drugs with a noted anti-cholinergic load such as antihistamines, olanzapine, furosemide, ranitidine, amitriptyline, digoxin, benztropine and oxybutynin – all contribute to mouth dryness. Some patients also experience dryness as a result of salivary gland dysfunction or mucosal changes due to radiotherapy, chemotherapy or previous surgery.

The simple provision of options such as soda water or pineapple or ginger beer ice blocks, the prompt treatment of oral thrush and vigilant lip care and oral mucosal moistening with artificial saliva or cool water are all mainstays of management.

Constipation

Constipation is a frequent and distressing problem in the elderly and in palliative care patients. In the palliative phase, the causes are usually a combination of opioid use, anti-cholinergic drug load, relative dehydration, low roughage intake, poor mobility, poor muscle strength, genetics, lifestyle and habit.

For many patients, reversible causes are not found. But all patients should be assessed for painful haemorrhoids and rectal fissures, as these can be simply treated. Earlier in the disease course, bulk-forming laxatives and high-fibre diets may be recommended. However, these treatments are generally contraindicated for palliative patients because these patients are unable to maintain the required fluid intake. Gentle (and regular) laxation can usually be achieved by means of the regular use of stool-softening drugs such as coloxyl and can be augmented by osmotic drugs such as glycol and, if necessary, the use of enemas.

Any patient receiving opiates should also be prescribed laxatives, and the constipating effects of opioids do not abate with prolonged use. Fentanyl and buprenorphine are both regarded as less constipating than morphine.

No aggressive management of constipation should occur before faecal impaction has been ruled out by a rectal examination. Impaction is when a hard mass of faeces forms in the rectum. Mucosal water absorption leads to progressive hardening of the mass, and patients may develop faecal fluid leak around the mass. If impaction is present, rectally administered stool softeners must accompany oral laxatives. In rare cases, patients may need manual disimpaction, which is an unpleasant procedure for all concerned. If monitoring is available, a low dose of subcutaneous or intranasal midazolam can provide relaxation and amnesia for the patient.

It is important to remember that constipation can be a symptom that heralds bowel obstruction, and severe and prolonged constipation can also cause true obstruction. Any patient with constipation and any evidence of abdominal pain, nausea or faecal fluid leak should be fully assessed with a rectal examination and abdominal x-ray. There have been cases of aggressive management of constipation in the context of undiagnosed bowel obstruction, leading to intestinal perforation. There have also been a few (thankfully rare) cases of overly aggressive laxative use leading to cardiac events as a result of severe electrolyte disturbance. Any patient who is presumed to be constipated but does not respond to appropriate treatment must therefore undergo imaging and examination, rather than simply being prescribed yet more medication.

Pressure sores

Palliative care patients are at extremely high risk of pressure sores (also known as bed sores, pressure ulcers and pressure areas) simply because they often have many of the known risk factors. These risk factors include being thin and wasted, having poor nutritional status, being bed-bound or unable to change position independently, and having poor skin integrity. Pressure sores can be extremely painful and are graded as to their severity. Initial changes are noted as red and tender areas, often over bony protuberances, and these can progress to skin loss and the development of ulcers. In extreme cases, underlying structures can be affected and lead to complications such as osteomyelitis (an infection of bone).

Once established, it is often impossible to heal pressure sores in unwell patients. The early instigation of pressure-relieving strategies is the most effective intervention, and this can often be facilitated by occupational therapy review. Patients and families need to be educated on the use of specialist pressure mattresses, foam chair inlays and padding. The patient should be assessed for other contributing factors, such as untreated fungal infections of the skin, urinary or faecal incontinence leading to skin irritation, and poor hygiene. A concern regarding the development of sacral pressure sores in a patient whose continence is managed with pads is, for instance, a valid reason for insertion of an indwelling catheter. Careful turning of unconscious or semi-conscious patients, and taking care to separate the knees and ankles with pillows and provide pressure relief for the ear, are examples of simple interventions that can prevent the development of painful lesions.

Wound care

In the advanced palliative phase of care, the usual aim of healing may simply not be possible. Malignant tissue does not scab, heal and form scars in the same way as normal tissue, and the bleeding, ooze and odour of malignant fungating wounds can prove challenging. Many patients are so distressed and embarrassed by their wounds that they withdraw from social interaction for this reason alone.

Appropriate dressings, on the advice of a specialist wound-care nurse if available, are the mainstay of treatment. Focus must always be maintained on patient comfort and dignity. Very wet lesions (such as fistula that leak large amounts of fluid) can be managed by placing a stoma bag over the lesion. The bag will not in any way aid healing, but this intervention can provide significant relief from the constant worry of managing a leaking wound. Similarly, the provision of charcoal-containing dressings and antibiotic-containing creams can assist in the management of malodorous wounds. Simple icing sugar or sugar paste dressings (not the flour-containing versions) are extremely effective for controlling odour.

Malignant wounds may potentially lead to catastrophic bleeding if they are eroding near a large vessel. The procedure used in normal wound care (applying pressure to allow the clotting cascade to control bleeding) may not be effective with the low platelet counts and altered skin homeostasis inherent in malignancy. It is therefore important to prepare the patient and family for the possibility of bleeding, and draw up a plan of action – including when to consider hospital transfer. Absorbent dressings and, in high-risk cases, adrenaline dressings may be required.

Adequate analgesia (including extra analgesia for dressing changes) is of course a vital part of palliative wound care.

Metastatic spinal cord compression

Expanding metastatic lesions in the spinal vertebrae can rapidly compress the spinal cord. Symptoms such as back pain, leg weakness and bladder and bowel changes should immediately lead to the consideration of metastatic spinal cord compression (MSCC) in any patient with a known malignancy.

High-dose steroid therapy and urgent radiation oncology review are vital because the longer the nerves are compressed, the less likely it is that functional recovery will occur.

Chapter 12

The good referral

Good referrals are all too rare. For any health practitioner who is asked to review a patient, the quality of the information in the referral is directly correlated with the quality of assessment and the relevance of advice given. In the palliative phase, it is even more important that referrals are thorough and appropriate.

The referral should always include the patient's age, sex and a brief review of the principal diagnosis. It is also vital to include a statement regarding disease extent and stage and functional level. The social circumstances of the patient (for example, living conditions, emotional support, availability of carers and any major interpersonal conflicts) and the main symptoms of concern should be highlighted, and the specific aim of review should be made clear.

Below are three examples of real referrals received by a tertiary palliative care service. All were asking for a review by a palliative care doctor for patients in the general medical wards of a large hospital:

'Thanks for seeing Mrs X. She is a 76-year-old woman with bowel cancer. Please see her regarding support at home.'

'Mr B is a 70-year-old man with stage 4 NSCLC (non small cell lung cancer) with mets to bone and liver. Wants to get home. Please review his pain.'

'Mrs M. is a palliative patient with bowel cancer. Thanks for seeing her.'

In contrast the following referral, while still quite brief, provides all the necessary information and gives the receiving practitioner a good idea of what is being requested:

'Thanks for seeing Bill T., a 69-year-old man with a 4-year history of heart failure. He has dilated cardiomyopathy and is maximally medically managed. Only just managing ADLs [activities of daily living] but house-bound on oxygen. Elderly wife just coping. Please see him to optimise management of breathlessness and with regard to palliative care support at home.'

In addition to providing the relevant information, it is also important to ensure that the language used is appropriate. The following referral may have been perfectly acceptable (indeed, very thorough) for a medical practitioner whose only aim was symptom control but was probably virtually indecipherable to the occupational therapist for whom it was intended:

'Mrs B, 49 yo F with stage 4 neuroendocrine lung c, mets liver, C4, L1, LVF only 30%, poor FEV1, O2 dependent Post ICU and inotropes now NFR. Pleural eff. Post VAT. Please see re mobility.'

For an occupational therapist, a far more appropriate referral for the same patient would have read:

'Thanks for seeing Mrs B, a 49-year-old lady with metastatic lung cancer. She has metastasis to the cervical and lumbar spine and is oxygen-dependent. Recently she was in the ICU [intensive care unit] and has had a pleuradesis [drain of pleural fluid], due to a pleural effusion. Lives with husband and now requires review regarding mobility and possible equipment at home.'

Careful and appropriate referral, and the provision of clear aims, will enable the clinician to optimise their contribution to patient outcome.

Pain

Pain is one of the most feared symptoms. For most tertiary palliative care units, it remains the number one reason for referral. Pain can have numerous causes, and can be both physical and psycho-spiritual. Practitioners should always accept that pain is 'whatever the patient says hurts', rather than whatever we (as healthcare workers) think should hurt.

Physical pain can range from the low-grade grumbling discomfort of osteoarthritis to the excruciating pain of peritonitis and everything in between. When we discuss or describe pain, it is useful to consider its site, character and pattern. Medical staff focus carefully on the description of pain. They have developed a large pain-specific vocabulary, but an accurate and unemotive description of the pain is appropriate for most situations. Good-quality information is imperative if management is to be optimal.

Saying 'Fred has such bad pain in his stomach that he's crying with it' may convey the severity of the situation but, for a practitioner trying to provide management, the information is too limited. However, 'Fred has very severe, intermittent, crampy pain in the middle of his abdomen' provides vital clues as to possible aetiology and therefore facilitates prescribing.

Information about the location of pain, and its pattern and character, is beneficial. Patients often find describing pain difficult but simple questions, such as 'Is it sharp or dull?', 'Does it come and go in waves or is it there all the time?' or 'Would you say it's more like the pain of sciatica or more like a toothache?', can provide a commonsense framework for communication. Grading systems (such as a scale of 1 to 10, with 10 being the 'worst pain imaginable') can be useful for assessing the effect of treatment.

The perception of pain is influenced by a number of factors, many of them not physical. A patient who, for example, watched a relative die in pain, who has experienced poorly controlled pain in the past, or who fears that worsening pain indicates that death is close, may seek to conceal the degree of their pain or may, conversely, experience pain with great severity. It is important always to consider the complete social and spiritual milieu of any patient for whom appropriate analgesia does not provide improvement. No amount of medication can manage the pain of significant psycho-spiritual distress, and referral to a pastoral care worker or a psychologist may be appropriate.

Just as pain may vary in site, pattern and character, so it can vary in aetiology and chronicity. Chronic degenerative lumbar pain is very different from the acute pain of a lumbar crush fracture. Information about the timeframe and onset of pain is helpful to prescribers. For example, it is inappropriate to manage chronic arthritis pain with opiates but the same medications are the management of choice in severe lumbar pain due to metastatic bone disease. Similarly, a good description can indicate whether a pain is likely to respond to anti-inflammatory medications or opiates, or whether there is likely to be a nerve pain component that may require adjuvant therapy.

Most healthcare practitioners are familiar with the concept of an 'analgesia ladder', which provides a visual model for escalating pain relief.

For many patients in the palliative phase of care, several steps of the ladder have probably occurred in the past, and adjuvant agents (such as dexamethasone, anti-depressants and anti-epileptics) are indicated. All medications have side-effects and analgesics are no exception, with dry mouth, constipation, nausea and confusion being common problems. Simple agents such as paracetamol should not be ignored even when opiate doses are significant, as they can still provide a valuable pain relief contribution. Paracetamol in appropriate doses is safe, even in the context of significant hepatic failure. For elderly, frail or very unwell patients, the liquid formulation is often preferable. At very high opioid doses, or if swallowing and 'pill burden' are an issue, paracetamol should be ceased.

The majority of patients will eventually require a background level of pain relief and many also require the addition of 'as needed' or 'breakthrough' medications to take when pain is exacerbated. Breakthrough pain occurs for many reasons, and sometimes without an obvious cause. Movement, abdominal peristalsis and positioning can all cause incidences of increased pain. The ideal breakthrough drug would have a very rapid onset and offset of action, as most 'breakthrough' pain is short-lived. It is often simpler, if possible, to use related medications for both background and 'as needed' dosing, although this may be problematic.

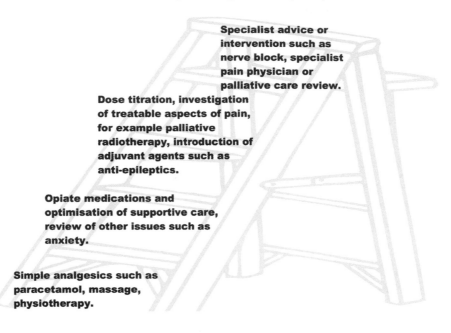

Specialist advice or intervention such as nerve block, specialist pain physician or palliative care review.

Dose titration, investigation of treatable aspects of pain, for example palliative radiotherapy, introduction of adjuvant agents such as anti-epileptics.

Opiate medications and optimisation of supportive care, review of other issues such as anxiety.

Simple analgesics such as paracetamol, massage, physiotherapy.

Figure 12.1 *The 'ladder of pain relief'*

It is important to identify the cause of pain exacerbations, and institute management strategies if possible. For most patients in the palliative phase, it is impossible to 'cure' the cause of pain. A physiotherapy or occupational therapy review regarding movement, support and modification may therefore be vital.

Patients and their families need to be educated regarding the use of analgesics, their side-effects and the role of 'as needed' doses. When it comes to pain relief, it is sometimes difficult to find a balance between extremes. On the one hand, a patient or family may refuse analgesia, despite distressing pain, due to fears of addiction or weakness. On the other hand, a patient or family may over-use analgesia for any minor discomfort. Thorough explanation and firm but gentle support are the bedrocks of management.

Healthcare staff need to explain carefully to patients what analgesia can, and cannot, be expected to achieve. It is inappropriate to promise perfect pain relief without side-effects to any patient:

'Bill, the pain in your back when you walk is due to the fact that the prostate cancer has invaded the bone and you now have lots of tiny breaks in there that we call 'micro fractures'. Whenever you move, they grate on each other, and that causes the pain. Unfortunately there is nothing we can do to fix that. It seems that the fentanyl patch keeps you very comfortable when you are resting but you will need to take extra doses of oxycodone when you walk. You'll always have a bit of discomfort but we can make sure that you are comfortable most of the time and that the pain when you walk is manageable.'

There are instances when pain is so severe that there needs to be an acceptance of side-effects, particularly drowsiness and immobility, for control to be gained. Patients with severe and difficult-to-control pain are usually admitted to hospital and, very occasionally, may require sedation. It is important to reassure patients with severe pain that these extreme options exist for management of pain in the terminal phase of life.

As the number of patients living for many years with slow-release opiate management of chronic pain increases, tertiary pain units are seeing increasing numbers of patients with difficult pain syndromes. Research indicates that long-term opiate use creates changes in cells that lead to increased perception of pain and decreased effectiveness of analgesics. Patients who experience a heightened degree of pain in response to unpleasant stimuli ('hyperalgesia') and patients who experience pain in response to benign stimuli ('allodynia') require assessment by a specialist pain team or palliative care team. These patients may require specialised adjuvant medications or may need to undergo 'opioid rotation', in which their analgesia medication is 'swapped' to another agent to improve control.

Radiotherapy remains the single most effective analgesic for isolated bone pain due to malignant disease for many patients. Single fraction radiotherapy can often be organised quickly, and even frail patients should be referred for review. The benefit occurs rapidly, lasts for months and has minimal or no side-effects.

More complex interventions for pain include nerve blocks and intra-thecal analgesia (in which pain medications are injected directly into the fluid that flows around the spinal cord). These are usually performed by anaesthetists or interventional radiologists, and patients in the palliative phase should be referred promptly.

For the majority of patients, a combination of slow-release and rapid-release opioid medication is effective in managing pain. Careful attention to side-effects and the provision of medications to manage nausea and constipation are vital. If side-effects become unacceptable, or if pain control is sub-optimal despite dose titration, opioid rotation may be very effective.

Rotation can be complex, and in most cases the dose equivalent of the new medication is reduced by 30–50% due to 'cross tolerance'. This is because pain is frequently more sensitive to a 'new' medication than it was to the 'old' medication. In this context, specialist advice is indicated. It is important to avoid a situation whereby a medication is simply increased without evidence of benefit. The result of this sort of careless prescribing can be patients on extremely high opioid doses who remain in pain and who require intensive pain management and the utilisation of specialist pain medications. A very small minority of patients, particularly those with a long history of illegal narcotic use, can develop very difficult-to-treat pain syndromes and seem resistant to the effects of most commonly used analgesics. These patients require referral to a tertiary unit.

Chapter 13
Grief and loss

When we love, we will grieve. Grief is a normal human emotion and, unpleasant as it is, there is no 'cure' for grief after the diagnosis of a life-limiting illness or the loss of a loved one. Many factors (including age, social support, pre-morbid coping mechanisms and psychological profile) affect our ability to return to a more normal pattern of functioning after a period of grief.

There is no standard measure that determines the 'normal' degree and duration of grief. The majority of parents who lose a child feel that they will 'never get over it'; yet most will recover to the point of being once again able to partake fully in life and enjoy interaction with loved ones. 'Pathological grieving' is said to be present when the expected degree and duration of grief is not followed, and when the person experiences severe retardation of their ability to function normally.

Elisabeth Kübler-Ross famously detailed five stages of grief, to which can be added concepts of initial numbness and avoidance, followed by intense and chaotic feelings of pain and later gradual reorganisation and reintegration. Current thinking tends to accept that grief may encompass all elements of this paradigm, or none of them, and that the experience of grief differs greatly from one person to another, and can only be understood on an individual basis (Kübler-Ross 2008). However, the experience of grief doesn't always follow a predictable course.

The duration of various elements of the grief process can vary widely. Healthcare workers may often experience difficult behaviour from families, carers or patients struggling with grief. It is inappropriate for any healthcare worker to be exposed to threatening, aggressive or insulting behaviour, but in many cases review of the processes of grief will enable the provision of appropriate support. Psychologists, psychiatrists, social workers and pastoral care workers can all make important contributions to grief management, and support should continue through the bereavement phase, which can take a variable length of time depending on the individual.

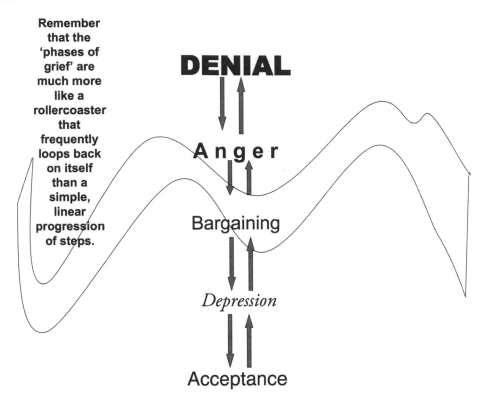

Remember that the 'phases of grief' are much more like a rollercoaster that frequently loops back on itself than a simple, linear progression of steps.

DENIAL

Anger

Bargaining

Depression

Acceptance

Figure 13.1 *The 'rollercoaster of grief'*

Healthcare workers, patients and families tend to be familiar with the concept of grief, but the concept of loss may be more difficult. Many patients describe their illness journey as a series of 'losses'. Initially, there may be the loss of confidence and income, later the loss of strength and independence, later again the loss of appetite, dignity and respect, and finally the loss of the ability to self-care and manage even the most basic functions. Finally, of course, there is the loss of loved ones as death occurs. The types and degrees of loss vary, depending on the age of the patient and their social circumstances. For some, the loss of the ability to mow the lawn is felt keenly, while others manage the fact that they can no longer deal with their own bowel motions with calm acceptance. Once again, the key factors in optimal management are individualised assessment and a willingness to accept, and act upon, the patient's own priorities.

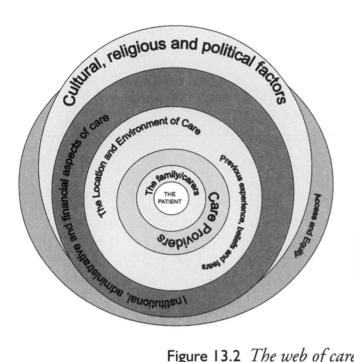

Optimal care provision relies on a complex web of inter-related and interdependent factors that no single individual or institution can control. Problems can occur at every level.

In many countries, for example, even simple opioid medications are not easily accessed. For other patients a fractured nuclear family may present a fundamental challenge.

Careful identification of the strengths, conflicts and weaknesses that surround each patient is a vital step towards developing a plan for optimal care at the end of life.

Figure 13.2 *The web of care provision*

Chapter 14
Caring for the carer

Working in palliative care can be incredibly rewarding. Just as it is possible to affect many people at the time of birth, so it is possible to have far-reaching effects at the time of death. For patients in the palliative phase of illness, small gains in comfort can have huge implications for quality of life. Families can be deeply affected by poor management of a loved one in the terminal phase. Similarly, dignified and effective management of symptoms in the very sick will be remembered for a long time and passed down through the generations. Healthcare providers in palliative care have an opportunity to provide compassionate and effective care for a highly vulnerable group of patients.

However, it can also be very stressful to care for patients who continue to become sicker and frailer and almost invariably die. Healthcare workers can develop 'burnout' without even being aware of what is happening to them. It is therefore imperative that any unit dealing with substantial numbers of palliative care patients has mechanisms in place to support staff and facilitate debriefing in a safe and supportive environment.

There are some nursing care issues that can only be truly appreciated by other nurses. Likewise, there are aspects of medical practice that can only be understood by other doctors. For example, it is unlikely that doctors will feel completely at ease discussing their feelings of frustration, stress or anxiety in an open forum. It may therefore be necessary to ensure that connections are made with suitable colleagues outside the unit.

Not all patients or their family members are likeable. Conversely, healthcare staff may closely identify with some patients, and feel great affection for them. Patients with particularly difficult symptom issues (such as fungating and malodorous wounds, necrotic mouth lesions or rectovaginal fistula) can prove challenging for staff to care for in an empathetic and dignified way.

The multidisciplinary team has an invaluable role in allowing safe and confidential discussion of these issues. All units should have a system by which any staff member can access support. There should also be a method of confidentially reporting any staff behaviour that is causing concern, and appropriate follow-up should be instigated. Appropriate breaks and holidays need to be taken, and a formal system of supported self-appraisal is paramount in ensuring that care delivery is sustainable.

Work within the palliative context can become very insular. Palliative care providers often feel that they are 'fighting a battle' against the wider healthcare system for the good of the patient and it is easy to develop a 'siege mentality'. This can lead to the assumption that palliative care practitioners always occupy the moral high ground, and that healthcare workers in other fields need correction. However, it is important to maintain perspective, and regular interaction with staff from other disciplines is beneficial. Quality control and practice audit processes aimed at reviewing procedures, combined with more informal self-reflection sessions, should be utilised to ensure that staff continue to 'look outwards' rather than focus solely on their own practice.

Chapter 15
Difficult discussions

The topic of euthanasia is difficult to avoid when discussing patients in the palliative phase but it is a basic tenet of the palliative care profession that euthanasia (or physician-assisted suicide) has no part in practice. It is not the role of this book to express an opinion on this topic.

It is reasonably common for doctors, in particular, to be asked to expedite the death of seriously ill patients. Families, patients and other healthcare workers frequently comment on the perception that the opiate doses used in palliative care shorten life. However, patients and their families can be assured that appropriate analgesia will not shorten life.

Research has indicated that, in the context of advanced and incurable illness, opiate doses (even at very high levels) do not shorten life but that poor symptom control, especially of pain, may (Portenoy, Sibirceva, *et al.* 2006). The cardiovascular and respiratory strain caused by severe pain is far greater than the impact of opiates on an opiate-tolerant physiology. Healthcare workers are often ill-informed regarding the use of opiates and sedatives at the end of life, and this can greatly increase anxiety at an already difficult time for patients, family and prescribers. It is far easier for a grieving family to blame 'the morphine' than to accept that a disease is the cause of death.

The 'law of double effect' is an oft-quoted ethical principal. It has four main elements:

- The nature of the act or intervention is good or, at worst, morally neutral.
- The intent behind the act or intervention is good.
- The good effect outweighs the bad effect, and the situation is sufficiently grave to allow acceptance of the bad effect.
- The agent of the act or intention exercises due diligence to minimise the bad effect.

The use of morphine to relieve pain in the terminal phase of life is the classic situation quoted to illustrate the principle of 'double effect'. It is acknowledged that increased morphine use in this context may present an identifiable risk of reducing respiratory rate, increasing drowsiness and increasing the chance of the development of a hypostatic pneumonia that may shorten life. However, the 'good effect' of morphine is the relief of pain and distress. In the final stage of life, it is accepted that the benefits of use outweigh the possible 'bad effects'.

In order to satisfy the legal, ethical and moral requirements of use in this situation, it is important that the doses are escalated only in response to the patient's symptoms, that the patient is appropriately monitored and cared for, and that the doses are reduced if the situation changes. In practice, this means that careful clinical documentation and actual patient review (as opposed to repeated telephone orders), are imperative.

The intent of a prescription is of critical importance – in the same way as the law considers someone who accidentally runs over a wayward pedestrian who runs in front of their car very differently from someone who intentionally uses their car to run over a person. If the intent is to give relief from pain and distress, the act is justifiable. However, if the intent is to shorten life then the act is legally, ethically and morally indefensible.

Studies have shown that the vast majority of patients who request euthanasia do so because they feel worthless, they are lonely, they feel they are a burden on loved ones, or because they want to spare their family and friends distress. The community perception is that patients request euthanasia due to uncontrolled pain but there is no evidence of this in studies that have been carried out in countries that support euthanasia and physician-assisted suicide.

High-dose analgesia and high-dose sedation (if required) are available in most wealthy countries to control pain, but patients who request termination of their lives are asking for something very different. Many patients demand the right to choose to die – simply because they would like to exert control over a situation that is, by its very nature, beyond their control. It is perhaps a human trait to wish to exert control even over death but healthcare workers who care for patients in the palliative phase of care need to become accustomed to working in a situation lacking in certainty. Furthermore, they need to develop the skills to assist patients, families and carers to function in this environment.

A careful and compassionate history, a firm and direct statement of what can, and cannot, be offered and an acknowledgement of uncertainty and fear are good starting points for discussion. It is important not to enter into any form of 'bargaining' with patients, and to ensure that information is provided truthfully and is not altered depending on the audience. Many patients fear that the 'waiting' for death will be prolonged and are relieved when the time to die approaches. The following conversation is based on a discussion with a real patient who requested euthanasia:

'I don't understand why you let patients suffer. Even dogs are treated better. They're put down and that's what I want. I just want to end it.'

'You're not a dog, Ted. I understand that you have pain and breathlessness due to the lung cancer. I think we can improve your pain control but it is important that you know that I will not do anything that will shorten your life.'

'Why the hell not? I want you to shorten it.'

'It is against the law for any person to knowingly shorten another person's life.'

'You would if it was you it was happening to. I should be able to have euthanasia if I want it. It would be a mercy.'

'No one has the right to have anything just because they want it, Ted. We will do everything we can to control the symptoms but I'm concerned that you feel so hopeless…'

'Why the hell wouldn't I feel hopeless? And you won't even help me…'

'I want to help you, but I will not kill you. I will give you some more pain relief and some medication to take away some of the anxiety and to try and take the edge off the depression…'

'I'm not **?!! depressed. I just want to die, that's all.'

'OK. Well, no one is in charge of that, neither you nor I, and I think that you will die over the next few weeks because the lung cancer is progressing very quickly. Our aim will be to make sure you are as comfortable as possible and that you can sleep when you want to until you die. Is that OK?'

'Well, it'll have to be, won't it? Because you're too lazy to let me die.'

'You're not asking me to let you die. You're asking me to knowingly shorten your life. It's called murder.'

'And you can't kill me because you're a bloody doctor…'

'Something like that… and we don't want doctors running around the place killing people, do we…'

'Hmmph. Well, you can make me sleep, can't you?'

Chapter 16
The angel at the end of the bed

Any review of palliative care literature will reveal a body of work dedicated to some very 'non-clinical' topics. Articles headed, for example, 'Palliative care nurses' perceptions of paranormal experiences', 'The role of a domestic cat in heralding impending death' and 'Deathbed visions' are frequently found in the literature. In many hospice units that care for dying patients, there are daily discussions of such topics. It is not the role of this book to pronounce on the existence or non-existence of spiritual phenomena, but it is important for practitioners to be open to a discussion of these issues with patients and carers.

'Deathbed visions' are well documented in historical and clinical literature (Longaker 2001, Rumbold 2004). They usually occur in the last hours or days of life and are associated with a delirium. Often, these visions are of previously deceased people known to the patient and they are widely thought to be a result of altered psychoactive chemicals due to 'brain failure' – in much the same way as urate and creatinine build up in cases of renal failure. They may sometimes be distressing and may occasionally be present in patients who do not exhibit any other signs of delirium. Patients with no other evidence of hallucination or misinterpretation of their environment may, quite matter-of-factly, state that they can see or speak to a deceased relative.

My own approach in such situations is 'never say never'. Patients are supported with medications such as haloperidol, the atypical anti-psychotics and sedation only if they are distressed. Challenging a dying person regarding the veracity of their experience is not beneficial, and family members should be supported in accepting that, for this person at this time, the experience is real.

Caring for patients during the palliative and terminal phases of illness is a great privilege. The opportunity to bestow care for its own sake alone is rare, especially in contemporary medical practice. An immeasurable difference can be made by small improvements to comfort in the terminal phase. By listening a great deal, asking a lot, acting a little and judging not at all, the palliative approach can provide optimal care as patients make the transition from the curative to the palliative paradigm and, ultimately, face their death.

Appendix
Case Studies

Patients' names have been changed in the following case studies.

Mr W. F.

Warwick was a 70-year-old man with a long history of smoking-related airway limitation. The previous year, he became increasingly short of breath and developed pleuritic (related to breathing, particularly inspiration) pain in the left chest. A computed tomography (CT) scan revealed a mass in the left hilar region. Bronchoscopy confirmed non-small cell lung cancer and he was commenced on a protocol of combined chemotherapy and radiotherapy. He tolerated therapy poorly and experienced vomiting, fatigue and dyspnoea (shortness of breath). His oncologist referred him to a palliative care clinic for review.

Warwick was very unhappy with the idea of referral and refused to attend the clinic. He changed both his oncologist and general practitioner, as he felt that referral to a palliative care clinic meant they had 'given up on him'. Over subsequent weeks, he was offered third-line chemotherapy at another centre but treatment was ceased after he developed neutropenia (a dangerous fall in his white blood cell count) and persisting nausea. His breathlessness was becoming more severe and he now had severe anorexia and cachexia.

He was subsequently admitted to a major hospital through the emergency department after collapsing at home. Review indicated that his electrolytes were deranged and that he was dehydrated. After fluid rehydration and the cessation of diuretics, his condition stabilised and discharge planning commenced. The following issues became clear:

- *Warwick had previously lived alone and had a son who lived several hours away and no other family.*
- *Friends had been concerned that he 'hadn't been coping' at home for several months.*
- *The condition of his home was described as 'filthy' and there was no food in the refrigerator.*

- *A telephone call to his general practitioner and the local pharmacy revealed that he was non-compliant with prescribed medications and did not turn up to scheduled visits.*

- *Formal mental state examination revealed dementia, with very poor short-term memory.*

- *Physiotherapy and occupational therapy review indicated that, although he could manage his own personal care, he required mobility aids, set up to eat and stand-by assistance for showering.*

- *Warwick's son, although concerned about his father, could not provide care, and agreed with the opinion that Warwick required placement in a care home for the elderly.*

After several arguments, during which Warwick threatened to self-discharge from hospital, the treating team referred him to pastoral care, social work and psychiatry. The psychiatry team agreed that he had dementia but did not find evidence of any mental health issue that required treatment. The social worker provided him with information regarding placement that he refused to accept and he refused to see the pastoral care worker.

Warwick was then referred to the palliative care clinical nurse. She reviewed him and found the following:

- *His shortness of breath was distressing and frightening.*

- *He was concealing and subsequently disposing of his prescribed sustained-release opiates, as he feared constipation.*

- *He was unable to sleep, due to hip and lumbar back pain.*

The nurse consulted with a palliative care doctor who reviewed Warwick and ordered x-rays and a bone scan. The doctor also found evidence of reflux oesophagitis on history and recommended antacid medications. The nurses spent time carefully and repeatedly explaining that the medications would help his breathing and nausea and that constipation could be managed by mild laxatives. He was subsequently commenced on a transdermal opiate to aid compliance. He was also prescribed liquid (rather than tablet) paracetamol, which he found more acceptable.

Imaging revealed a lytic metastatic lesion in lumbar vertebrae 2 and 3 and a similar lesion in the left hip. After discussion with his son, Warwick was referred to radiation oncology with simple and careful explanation regarding the role of treatment for pain relief. He had a single fraction of treatment to each area, with benefit.

Warwick was eventually placed in an elderly care home. His transdermal opiate dose was titrated in the hope of improving his dyspnoea but he remained very short of breath on any activity. The introduction of 'as needed' morphine syrup proved very beneficial. The staff ensured careful compliance with his bowel-care regime, as any sign of constipation resulted in refusal to accept analgesia. He was subsequently commenced on a nocturnal dose of a mood-stabilising medication to assist with his night-time confusion and agitation. His son agreed with a plan of comfort-only care and Warwick died peacefully four months later.

When the care team reviewed Warwick's case they noted the following points:

- *Identification of dementia is a vital step in patient management. It facilitates involvement of the next of kin or surrogate decision-maker, optimises communication and guards against potentially unsafe outcomes such as discharging patients without suitable supervision and compliance aids.*

- *There is no substitute for a careful history and examination. For example, confusing simple 'reflux' with more complex disease or therapy-related nausea can lead to poor symptom control.*

- *Compliance can only be optimised once the care team has identified patient-centred issues such as, in this case, the fear of constipation.*

- *Careful and repeated explanation that connects the proposed medication or intervention to the symptom is an important step towards compliance.*

Ms H. B.

Helena was a 58-year-old single woman who was diagnosed with glioblastoma multiforme (an aggressive form of brain tumour) after she became confused and had a seizure. She underwent surgery and the tumour in the right frontal area of her brain was debulked. She subsequently underwent whole-brain radiotherapy and managed very well for two months.

Unfortunately, however, she experienced a recurrence of the headaches, dysarthria (slow, slurred and difficult to understand speech) and seizures that heralded her initial diagnosis. It became clear that her disease had returned. Dexamethasone (a steroid medication) was recommenced at a high dose with excellent response. She remained well for a further two weeks before her symptoms once again became disabling and she was admitted to hospital. The radiation oncology team stated that no more treatment could be offered, and the neurosurgical team did not feel that further surgery was possible. Helena and her niece were dissatisfied with this and she discharged herself against advice. Subsequently she underwent further debulking surgery at another centre and was treated with one fraction of targeted radiotherapy.

Helena was referred for palliative care review one week after surgery and was noted to be drowsy and confused, incontinent of both faeces and urine, unable to mobilise and requiring high-level care. Her niece Penny was distressed, as she felt guilty that further surgery had been attempted, despite advice that the risks were very high. The therapeutic alliance with the radiation oncology team had broken down completely during previous admissions when Penny had accused the team of refusing to treat her aunt with more radiation because they had 'given up on her and didn't care' and had threatened litigation.

103

Helena had therefore been admitted by the general medical team on call and they had repeated her head scan. This found, as expected, disease recurrence and significant surrounding oedema, with some bleeding. Her blood tests were unremarkable. Increased dexamethasone had failed to improve Helena's functional state.

The palliative care doctor and nurse reviewed the notes, examined Helena and met with her niece and the niece's husband. The doctor involved sought information from both medical and radiation oncology teams and the nurse collected detailed information about Helena's nursing care on the ward. The following picture emerged:

- Helena required care for all activities of daily living. She needed sling lifter transfers and feeding.

- She communicated in single words but her responses were inconsistent and she intermittently followed only simple commands.

- Seizures had been controlled by medication but Helena was experiencing episodes of confusion and drowsiness. However, at other times, she could appear more alert and would attempt to sit up and would interact with visitors.

- Helena had cared for her sister, who had suffered from depression, for many years and had acted as a mother to her sister's only child.

- As a result, her niece Penny felt a huge debt of gratitude to Helena and was devastated to be losing her. She had always hoped that Helena would serve as a grandmother to her children.

- The doctors involved felt that, if an acute event (such as an infection or clot) did not occur, Helena could live for many months but that there was no chance of meaningful functional improvement.

- Helena's care needs were such that she required nursing home placement but, due to her age, the process was slow and laborious.

- Penny felt guilty about 'putting her in a home' and was noted to be repeatedly 'force-feeding' her aunt high-protein supplements, and trying to sit her up in bed without proper assistance. Penny had complained about the lack of physiotherapy being provided.

- The ward staff felt the niece was 'in denial' about Helena's condition and they found Penny rude and demanding.

The palliative care team met formally with Penny on two occasions, with the specific aim of informing her about Helena's disease state. They affirmed the challenges presented by brain tumours that have such devastating consequences but often leave the rest of a patient's body relatively unscathed. They discussed the fluctuating levels of alertness and communication, and emphasised that this was commonly seen in this form of cancer. They also explained that the effect of dexamethasone, whilst initially apparently 'miraculous', was temporary. They encouraged

Penny and her husband to express their concerns and questions, and answered them as simply and accurately as possible.

The team involved a pastoral care worker who was able to encourage Penny to acknowledge the huge debt of gratitude she felt to her aunt, and to explore the resurgent feelings about her own unhappy childhood that her aunt's illness had provoked. The pastoral care worker acknowledged the multiple losses that Penny had suffered and told her that the loss of 'a potential future' was a valid reason to grieve. Penny was subsequently able to acknowledge her deep desire to 'keep her aunt with her', despite a growing realisation that her condition was irreversible and would end in death.

Despite initial reluctance on the part of the ward staff, Penny was encouraged to assist in the day-to-day care of her aunt, including hygiene tasks. Although this process was initially difficult and stressful, it provided experiential proof of the magnitude of Helena's care needs. Penny was then able to accept that rehabilitation was not possible and that nursing home placement was required.

The team subsequently commenced the processes involved in placement. After a further six weeks in hospital, Helena was placed in a nursing home. The palliative care outreach team offered support to the nursing home, and the pastoral care worker had intermittent but continuing contact with Penny. The general practitioner now caring for Helena declined further input from the palliative care team until the terminal phase of illness, when an infusion containing morphine and clonazepam was commenced.

Penny continues to be followed up by the pastoral care team, who feel she is at a high risk of a pathological bereavement process. They have requested formal review by a psychologist due to concerns that she may suffer a major depressive episode.

When the case was reviewed, the following points were emphasised:

- Care teams need to provide careful, consistent and repeated explanation of symptoms to concerned family members. For example, it would have been very beneficial to have explained the fluctuating course of many brain tumour patients, and the initially impressive but only transient effects of dexamethasone, earlier in Helena's disease journey.

- It is important that the team constantly remembers to ask themselves 'What are the family/ carers feeling?' It is easy for experienced clinicians to forget that the transient improvement that we see as a medication effect can be interpreted by laypeople as evidence of recovery.

- Good nursing care is a major therapeutic intervention that is often undervalued. Some family members need direct experience of the burden of care before they can appreciate the issues involved.

- The understandable desire to withdraw from interacting with a family member as soon as it becomes 'difficult' must be avoided. If a room becomes 'difficult' to enter, it is precisely *the room that you should go into twice! Silence and avoidance will only worsen already strained communication and will feed feelings of anger, discrimination and paranoia. Often, the recruitment of a team member not previously involved in the tension can be very beneficial.*

Mr B. P.

Bill was a 92-year-old man with moderate Alzheimer's-type dementia who had lived in a local nursing home for 12 years. After several months of fatigue, weight loss and intermittent abdominal pain, he was taken to the emergency department following the passage of a large amount of black stool (malaena) and a collapse. He required intravenous (IV) fluid resuscitation and was transfused with three units of packed red blood cells. A CT scan confirmed the clinical findings of a mass in the left lower quadrant of the abdomen, and a presumptive diagnosis of bowel cancer was made. He was noted to have metastatic disease in his liver.

Bill subsequently underwent a bone scan and was found to have several metastatic lytic lesions in his pelvis. It was decided that biopsy would require a colonoscope and would not change management and it was not performed. Due to his widespread disease, chemotherapy was not an option and Bill was commenced on regular paracetamol, a mild laxative and low-dose sustained-release morphine. He was discharged back to the nursing home.

Bill's family consisted of two sons and a daughter, and multiple grandchildren and great-grandchildren. His family simply wanted him to be kept comfortable and elected his eldest daughter, Pearl, to be their delegate. Pearl met with the nursing home staff and detailed an advance care directive (living will), which stipulated that Bill was not for cardiopulmonary resuscitation, not for intubation or intensive care admission, and was to be kept at the nursing home and provided with comfort-only care in the event of deterioration.

He managed well for several months and continued to enjoy visits from his family and attend activities in the nursing home. He experienced the occasional passage of rectal blood-stained mucus and wore a pad. His left hip pain worsened and he was referred to a radiation oncologist for review. After initial family reluctance, he was treated with one fraction of palliative radiotherapy to the hip, with excellent response.

Four months after diagnosis, it was noted that Bill was becoming more frail and forgetful. His appetite was minimal and he was spending large amounts of time asleep. His family accepted his deterioration as part of his cancer and remained happy with the plan for comfort-only care. However, one Saturday night, Bill collapsed and had a large-volume rectal bleed. Overnight staff at the nursing home was minimal, and the relatively inexperienced staff present felt unable to manage the situation. Bill was therefore transferred by ambulance to the nearest emergency department. His family was informed of events and, although she was initially annoyed, Pearl said she understood the reasons for transfer.

Over subsequent days, Bill's condition slowly improved and discharge was planned. He returned to the nursing home (requiring high-level nursing care) but was generally comfortable and settled. He was now spending the majority of his time in bed and required assistance for hygiene and feeding. He experienced another significant rectal bleed and was, once again, transferred to the emergency department.

Palliative care review was requested by the emergency department staff and Pearl articulated her frustration about her father's situation by saying that she felt that 'The emergency department staff don't want him because he's palliative, and the nursing home don't want him because they're scared he's going to bleed to death before their eyes.' Bill was transfused 2 units of blood in an effort to improve the breathlessness resulting from anaemia, without noticeable benefit. Pearl decided that he was not to undergo further transfusion.

A nurse from the palliative care team travelled to the nursing home in order to fully understand the issues from their point of view. The following points were noted:

- *Bill was a much-loved resident and there was a strong desire to care for him to the end of his life.*

- *Staffing, particularly overnight, was minimal, with only one registered nurse for 64 residents. The majority of staff were young and/or inexperienced aids in nursing.*

- *Palliative care outreach staff were not able to administer medications to nursing home patients on site, and only senior nurses (clinical nurse consultants) were permitted to visit.*

- *The possibility of a catastrophic rectal bleed causing Bill's death was something that the nursing staff felt unqualified to manage. There was significant fear around this issue.*

- *The general practitioner caring for Bill, although willing to chart medications to be used in the case of a terminal event, did not feel that the nursing home would be able to manage a large-volume bleed leading to death.*

- *Further to this, it became clear that legislation prevented the provision of stat (immediate) doses of subcutaneous agents, such as morphine and midazolam, in the nursing home, by nursing home staff.*

In view of the information gathered, it became clear that, although everyone wanted Bill to be cared for in his nursing home, this was not possible. The other care options were explained: remaining in the acute hospital setting, being transferred to a hospice, or being cared for at home. Much to the surprise of the care team, Pearl elected to care for her father at home, with the support of her husband and daughter.

Bill was reviewed by the occupational therapist, and equipment (including a hospital bed, a commode and an oxygen concentrator) was organised. An indwelling urinary catheter was placed to simplify Bill's care. The palliative care doctor and registrar carefully explained to Pearl and her daughter the medication regime and the use of 'as needed' breakthrough analgesia. They reiterated that a catastrophic bleed would be sudden and visually confronting and confirmed, as far as possible, that the family were prepared to deal with this eventuality. Palliative care outreach was organised to visit Bill and Pearl daily. Luckily it was possible to provide a single drawn-up syringe of morphine, for use only in case of a terminal event.

Two weeks after going home, Bill did experience a massive rectal bleed. He died before the palliative care outreach staff could attend and before Pearl had a chance to administer any medication. The service had provided green towels that mask the appearance of blood but, despite this, the volume of blood lost was confronting. Pearl and the other family members coped with the experience with a great degree of serenity and acceptance, and were justifiably proud of the care they had provided for Bill in the final stages of his life.

Pearl was followed up by the bereavement support service of the palliative care unit and was specifically asked if she experienced any post-traumatic effects from her father's death. She stated that, although she did of course think about the event, she was not distressed by the memory at all. On review of this case, the following points were noted:

- Some families cope with things incredibly badly. Others cope with extreme challenges incredibly well. It's difficult to predict in advance which way a family will react.

- The presumption that 'being in a nursing home' is always a solution to care is, at least in Australia, naive. Nursing home patients have extremely high care needs but staffing is often sub-optimal and poorly supported. The organisation and governance of these facilities often makes care provision by outside providers impossible.

- For many families, the fact that they provided care (even if only for a few days) for a loved one at home is a source of great comfort during bereavement. Even if the care team feel there is a high likelihood of terminal 'care at home' failing, families should be allowed the opportunity to try if they wish.

Mr N. F.

Ned was an 82-year-old man initially referred to the palliative care service for support at home. He had a diagnosis of squamous cell cancer that had first occurred in his throat eight years previously. He had undergone extensive surgery and radiotherapy in the past, and had recently been noted to have metastatic disease in his liver.

Ned had been widowed two years earlier, and still missed Jean (his 'wife and soulmate of 60 years') dreadfully. They had never had children and Ned had no other family. He lived alone in a small, cluttered home in a rural town.

The palliative care outreach service visited Ned initially to assist in the management of pain and constipation. His symptoms improved but his general condition continued to deteriorate gradually, with progressive fatigue, weight loss and weakness. A local recurrence of his disease had begun to cause progressive dysphagia (difficulty swallowing) and he could now manage only soup and custard. Ned was referred to a surgeon by his family doctor to discuss a feeding tube but he declined, stating that the trip to the teaching hospital was too much for him and that he had no appetite for food anyway.

Over several weeks, Ned's opiate dose increased. He became myoclonic (involuntary, coarse jerking movements) and a blood test revealed that his kidney function was much worse than it had previously been. His analgesia was changed from morphine-based to fentanyl-based, with improvement. The nurses visiting Ned began to notice that he really wasn't managing at home and that he had begun to call the service very frequently. The combination of the post-surgical and post-radiation changes, and the disease recurrence, resulted in difficulty swallowing, dribbling of offensive-smelling saliva and very difficult-to-understand speech. As a result of these issues, Ned refused to allow friends to visit and stopped going to town. He also became unable to make himself understood on the telephone and was fearful that he would be unable to call for help if needed. He refused his family doctor's offer of admission to the small local health centre, as he didn't want 'those girls having to wash me'.

For several weeks, it was presumed that Ned would refuse admission to any service, and that offering hospice admission two hours away in a large centre would, of course, be declined. However, this was not the case. A new palliative care registrar called to see Ned at home and offered him a hospice bed. Ned gratefully accepted it and immediately began packing. He was transferred to the unit by ambulance the next day, after delivering a copy of his final will and testament to the executor of his estate, the local publican.

Ned died in the hospice four weeks later. His symptoms were managed by a subcutaneous infusion of fentanyl and metoclopramide. Episodic use of metronidazole suppositories assisted in the management of oral odour, and he required only minimal sedation in the last two days of his life.

His case is notable not for the difficulty of his symptoms, but for how much he enjoyed his admission to the hospice. He quickly became a favourite of the nurses, cleaners and kitchen staff. He was provided with the daily papers and wheeled out into the sun most mornings to watch the traffic and everyone enjoyed stopping by his room for a brief chat, even though it was often very difficult to understand him. He received physiotherapy for his legs, even though he was by now unable to walk, simply because he enjoyed the attention. His birthday was marked by cards and cake and singing. When he died, there was a genuine outpouring of grief.

Ned taught the unit a lot about the palliative approach to care. For him, dying was not the problem and his physical symptoms could be managed adequately. For Ned, it was loneliness and the need to preserve his dignity that mattered most. The palliative approach to care enabled the focus to be placed on Ned as a person, rather than on Ned as a cancer patient. As a result, he experienced an optimal terminal phase of care.

Mr E.C.

Eddy was a 70-year-old man with a long history of personality disorder. In his younger days, he was noted to have undertaken frequent risk-taking behaviour, had used excessive amounts of alcohol and had been jailed several times for burglary. More recently, his health had deteriorated, with alcohol-related liver disease, high blood pressure, insulin-dependent type 2 diabetes and a slowly progressive dementia that was considered to be of mixed aetiology. Over six months, Eddy had begun experiencing increased episodes of paranoia and no reversible cause for this was found. He was subsequently placed in a low-care hostel and managed quite well for several months.

Over recent days, Eddy had begun refusing his medications and accusing the hostel staff of trying to poison him. Palliative care review was requested. The consultation documentation made specific mention of the provision of subcutaneous or intravenous 'management of paranoia and verbal aggression and the provision of effective sedation' as the primary aim of the consultation.

On examination, Eddy was observed to be agitated and paranoid. He was noted to have worsening jaundice, and further questioning revealed that he had stopped using his lactulose. On further physical examination (which was difficult), he was noted to have severe oral thrush.

Eddy was subsequently treated with anti-psychotic agents and intermittent oral, low-dose sedatives, followed by aggressive management of his oral thrush. The alteration in food taste caused by the thrush (which he had interpreted as 'poisoning') abated and compliance improved. Eddy began to accept regular lactulose and his condition improved for several weeks. He died in hospital four weeks later, after developing pneumonia.

This case is notable for two reasons. Firstly, once again, careful physical examination and history held the clues that led to appropriate management. Secondly, if the aim of the consultation request had been followed without due care, it is likely that Eddy's life would have been significantly shortened. Any request to sedate a patient needs to be considered very carefully. Why is the request being made? Why is it being made now? And does the patient's best interest remain at the centre of the request? For some patients reaching the end of life, sedation is an effective tool for the management of distress, but for patients like Eddy there is a risk of it being used as an easier, and inappropriate, alternative. Sedating Eddy would have greatly increased his already high risk of complications such as hypostatic ('not moving') pneumonia, aspiration (due to inhaling food or saliva), pneumonia and deep vein thrombosis, any of which would have had a high probability of resulting in his death.

Further reading and references

Abernethy, A.P., Currow, D.C., Frith, P., Fazekas, B.S. *et al*. (2003). Randomised, double blind, placebo controlled crossover trial of sustained release morphine for the management of refractory dyspnoea. *British Medical Journal*. **327**, 523.

Abernethy, A.P., McDonald, C.F., Frith, P.A., Clark, K. *et al*. (2010). Effect of palliative oxygen versus room air in relief of breathlessness in patients with refractory dyspnoea: a double-blind, randomised controlled trial. *The Lancet*. **376** (9743), 784–93.

Bruera, E. & Yennurajalingam, S. (2012). Palliative care in advanced cancer patients: how and when. *Oncologist*. **17** (2), 267–73.

Caraceni, A., Hanks, G., *et al*., European Palliative Care Research Collaborative (EPCRC) & European Association for Palliative Care (EAPC). (February 2012). Use of opioid analgesics in the treatment of cancer pain: evidence-based recommendations from the EAPC. *Lancet Oncology*. **13** (2), e58–68.

Caresearch. http://www.caresearch.com.au/Caresearch/Default.aspx Online palliative care information resource.

Casciato, D.A. & Territo, M.C. eds. (2012). *The Manual of Clinical Oncology*. Philadelphia: Lippincott Williams and Wilkins.

Doyle, D., Hanks, G., Cherny, N.I. & Calman, K. eds. (2003). *Oxford Textbook of Palliative Medicine*. New York, USA: Oxford University Press.

Groves, R. & Klauser, H. (2005). *The American Book of Dying*. Berkeley, California, USA: Celestial Arts Publishing.

Jennings, A.L., Davies, A.N., Higgins, J.P.T., Gibbs, J.S.R. & Broadley, K.E. (2003). A systematic review of the use of opioids in the management of dyspnoea. *British Medical Journal*. **327**, 523.

Kübler-Ross, E. (2008). *On Death and Dying*. London: Routledge Publishing, Taylor & Francis Group.

Longaker, C. (2001). *Facing Death and Finding Hope: A Guide to the Emotional and Spiritual Care of the Dying*. New York, USA: Broadway Books.

Portenoy, R.K., Sibirceva, U., *et al*. (2006). Opioid use and survival at the end of life: a survey of a hospice population. *Journal of Pain Symptom Management*. **32** (6), 532–40.

Rumbold, B. (2004). *Spirituality and Palliative Care*. New York, USA: Oxford University Press.

Saunders, C. (1990). *Hospice and Palliative Care: An Interdisciplinary Approach*. London: Hodder Arnold.

Twycross, R. & Wilcock, A. eds. (2011). *Palliative Care Formulary (PCF4)*. Nottingham, UK: Palliativedrugs.com Ltd.

Twycross, R., Wilcock, A. *et al*. (2009). *Symptom Management in Advanced Cancer*. Nottingham, UK: Palliativedrugs.com Ltd.

Wilber, K. & Wilber, T. (2001). *Grace and Grit: Spirituality and Healing in the Life and Death of Treya Killam Wilber*. Boston, Massachusetts, USA: Shambala Publications.

Wolfe, J., Hinds, P. & Sourkes, B. (2011). *Textbook of Interdisciplinary Pediatric Palliative Care*. Philadelphia, USA: Saunders, Elsevier Group.

Index